UP

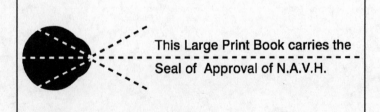

This Large Print Book carries the
Seal of Approval of N.A.V.H.

UP

HOW POSITIVE OUTLOOK CAN TRANSFORM OUR HEALTH AND AGING

HILARY TINDLE, M.D., M.P.H.

THORNDIKE PRESS
A part of Gale, Cengage Learning

GALE
CENGAGE Learning·

Detroit • New York • San Francisco • New Haven, Conn • Waterville, Maine • London

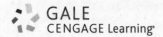

Thorndike Press® Large Print Health, Home & Learning.
The text of this Large Print edition is unabridged.
Other aspects of the book may vary from the original edition.
Set in 16 pt. Plantin.

LIBRARY OF CONGRESS CATALOGING-IN-PUBLICATION DATA

Tindle, Hilary.
    Up : how positive outlook can transform our health and aging / by Hilary Tindle, M.D. M.P.H. — Large print edition.
        pages cm
    Originally published: New York, New York : Hudson Street Press, 2013.
    Includes bibliographical references and index.
    ISBN 978-1-4104-6306-7 (hardcover) — ISBN 1-4104-6306-0 (hardcover) 1. Health behavior. 2. Positive psychology. 3. Aging—Psychological aspects. 4. Large type books. I. Title.
    RA776.9.T53 2013b
    613—dc23   2013025549

Published in 2013 by arrangement with Hudson Street Press, a division of Penguin Group (USA)

Printed in the United States of America
1 2 3 4 5 6 7 17 16 15 14 13

*For my parents, Matt, our daughters,
and everyone who has shown me
how to find life in the desert*

CONTENTS

1
HOW OUR OUTLOOK DRIVES OUR HEALTH AND AGING

"I wonder how many times you almost died?" my father asked me while we waited for our food at the Greek diner Salonica on Fifty-seventh Street, at the edge of the University of Chicago campus. In my third year of college, a previously undiagnosed congenital heart condition came crashing into my life and set me on a path to explore the attitudes that I now view as some of the most basic building blocks of health and disease. The gravity of my condition crystallized during the first week after successful cardiac surgery, and my father finally felt safe enough to pose this obvious question. There had been several times during my childhood when I had come close to collapsing, but every one of these mishaps had followed episodes of intense exertion, like running a three-hundred-yard dash in grade school or climbing out of the Grand Canyon as a high school student. Consequently, I had always passed them off as "overdoing it," and sometimes didn't even mention them to anyone. My dad and I reflected on the events of the past few months: The previous summer, my energy level had inexplicably taken a dive. One Sunday morning while having dim sum with friends in Chinatown, I had dropped a full glass of water — completely forgetting that my hand was supposed to be holding it — sending it clanking over the porcelain dishes and dumplings and shattering on the floor. I had even fallen asleep during my medical school entrance exams, waking up drooling over the biology section.

Having scarcely completed adolescence, it did not even occur to me that there could be something *really* wrong. But after several weeks involving similar incidents, I thought I may have mononucleosis and finally made an appointment at the student health center. After hearing my story, the internist detected a loud heart murmur and immediately shipped me off to get a cardiac ultrasound. In the dark, quiet viewing rooms of the echocardiography suite, there were raised eyebrows as successively senior cardiologists were called in to help interpret the results. I looked at the shadowy pictures of my beating chambers with suspense and intrigue, as if they were part of an exciting movie. Not until years later would I realize that my state of general wonder throughout this process — peppered though it was with fear and doubt — would help preserve my sanity through the events that followed. I did not yet know how to read an echocardiogram, and could not discern the mass of tissue in the middle of the heart chamber called the left ventricle. The mass was partially attached to the mitral valve — the valve bisecting the left atrium (top chamber) and the left ventricle (bottom chamber). The walls of the left ventricle had become hypertrophied, or thickened, because of the very high pressure required to pump blood through the mass and out to the rest of my body. My heart had reached a point where it was simply no longer able to perform. I needed major surgery as soon as possible.

After the initial shock and uncertainty, I became "the little patient that could." I put the surgery date on my calendar and told my relatives, friends, professors, and classmates. I met with my cardiac surgeon, the late Dr. Robert Karp, and asked him a list of twenty-two questions I had typed out on my PC, everything from how long the surgery would take (two to three hours) to the likelihood of dying on the table (5 percent or less). My final question — "Is there anything that I can do as a patient to make your job as a doctor easier?" — produced the first grin I'd seen on him yet. "You already have," he told me. I didn't catch his meaning then, but now as a practicing physician I know what it's like to work with a genuinely motivated patient, and I understand why he smiled at me. My upbeat attitude made me an easier patient to treat, someone willing to adhere to his medical advice and to do my part to attain the best possible outcome. That didn't mean I wasn't afraid. In fact, my concern about dying on the table prompted a couple of urgent visits to student mental health services: I didn't want to go to my grave with too much unfinished business. Within a couple of weeks I was on the operating table while Dr. Karp cut open my left atrium, reached across my mitral valve, and sliced away the offending blob.

After a brief ICU stay and four more days on the cardiac floor, I walked out of the hospital into a sharp Chicago December wind, leaning half of my body weight on each of my parents. Now on the mend, with a fresh scar traversing my chest, I basked in the warmth of my circumstances — hot Greek food, the love of my mom and dad, support of friends and professors, and the impeccable skill of my surgeon and his team, all culminating in the miracle of my being able to sit up without assistance. I had been given a second chance, and I was ecstatic to be alive.

The very experience of having felt so weak after surgery, in which it took real effort on some mornings to even hold my head up, allowed me a glimpse of frailty that most twenty-year-olds never get. Ironically, feeling close to my own mortality provided a rare and valuable reference point that only bolstered my hopefulness. During open heart surgery, my heart stopped beating for two hours on bypass, but I woke *up* — knowing that every day is a gift and that it is possible to overcome the most dire of situations. Looking back twenty years later from the vantage point of an NIH-funded academic physician, wife, and mother, I realize now it was the first time a serious situation had forced my "outlook" hand, and, instinctively, I played the hope card. This somewhat unconscious act, as well as the positive outcome itself — a 360-degree spin from healthy young woman to invalid and back again — began the evolution of the can-do attitude that often becomes my default. This outlook kicks in at two a.m., overriding all circadian rhythms, when I'm on call and paged to the bedside of a patient who has just gone into cardiac arrest. It helps me visualize an ill person becoming well again, even before he heals, because having witnessed the "other side," I know what proper care and tending can do for the human body. Above all, it fans the voice inside my head that declares things will eventually change, often for the better, even when the specifics remain uncertain.

Our outlook — a term I have chosen to describe our unique patterns of thinking, feeling, and interacting with ourselves and with the world — fundamentally impacts our health and aging. Outlook encompasses our personality, character traits, general disposition, and attitudes, all of which are words used by researchers and clinicians to describe our psychological makeup. While I use many of these terms interchangeably, I decided on the umbrella term *outlook* for several reasons. First, we can relate to it on a gut level: Our outlook is the lens through which we view the world. Unlike other terms, which carry connotations of permanence, outlook allows for the possibility of something new — as in "gain a new outlook on life." This is key, because *Up* is not an academic discussion of the psychological

14

underpinnings of aging, although I do include as much of the research as I can fit in. *Up* invites you to take a personal inventory — and, if necessary, to make changes geared toward maximizing your health at any age.

When we deconstruct our outlook into its nuts and bolts — the unique patterns of thinking and feeling that drive so much of our lives — we begin to see it from a different perspective. We begin to see not only *why* our outlook may lead us to decisions and behaviors but also *where* we may want to tweak it in the service of our own healthy aging, and *how* to undertake this change. Our outlook, research shows, has the potential to influence every facet of our health, from how quickly we recover from an illness or surgery to whether we become depressed, develop cardiovascular risk factors, or suffer a heart attack, stroke, or cancer, and even how well we care for ourselves when our health begins to break down.

Aspects of outlook — such as the character trait of optimism, defined by research psychologists as the general expectation of good things to come — have also been linked to longevity. Results from a study my colleagues and I published in the journal

Circulation (August 2009) on almost one hundred thousand American women showed that middle-aged and older female optimists, compared with pessimists (people who have a generally negative expectation of the future), were less likely to smoke or have diabetes, high cholesterol, high blood pressure, symptoms of depression, and obesity; they were also more physically active. Optimists lived *healthier* and *longer* lives than pessimists, exhibiting a 16 percent lower risk of a first heart attack and a 30 percent lower risk of death from heart disease by the end of the study. In these same women we studied another character trait, called cynical hostility, which is a type of anger involving a deep mistrust of other people. This mistrust stems from the belief that most people are selfish, dishonest, and unworthy. Women who had the highest levels of cynical hostility, compared with those with the lowest levels, were 16 percent more likely to die over eight years of study follow-up.

My research joins the growing ranks of findings from around the world that point in the same direction: A positive outlook is good medicine. Two decades of clinical practice as an internist have brought me to the same conclusion, demonstrating repeatedly how outlook provides some people with the gumption to seize opportunities, and in other cases seems to sabotage any hope of healing. In fact, very soon after I began my formal research training, I realized that the body of evidence was pointing to something bigger than any one disease or any one subgroup of patients. *Everyone* owns an outlook. And the truth is, we may have more control over our outlook than anything else. My clinical practice and early research spurred me to ask some pivotal questions that hold the promise of an exciting new reason to look *up:* **If our outlook is associated with a higher risk of aging-related diseases such as heart attack, stroke, cancer, and death itself, is it associated with aging, period? Does an unhealthy outlook make us older faster? And does a healthy outlook actually keep us physiologically younger?**

THE SCIENCE OF OUTLOOK AND AGING

Aging has become a loaded term these days — walk into any mall or search the Internet and you'll be greeted with a dizzying array of antiaging products purporting to turn back the clock and make you look and feel younger. But in strictly medical terms, healthy aging is defined as growing older while steering clear of mental and physical disability, and the field has become a major medical frontier. In fact, aging experts now have a term for living healthily to a ripe old age: *compression of morbidity.* What it means is that, ideally, we "compress" as much of our disease and disability as possible into the very last little bit of our life, so that we remain lucid and able-bodied enough to enjoy as much time as we can prior to our demise. Or as my colleagues who are aging experts say, "Live a long and healthy life — then fall off the cliff." Following this advice means paying as much attention, if not more, to our *health span* as to our *life span.*

So aging is much broader than the white-haired, wrinkled, cane-toting physical and mental debility most people associate with "getting old." The process actually takes place on multiple levels, every second of every day. For simplicity's sake, we can divide aging into three main categories: visible outward changes such as wrinkles and stooped posture; telltale variations in our organs such as atrophy of the brain, meaning loss of neurons; and microscopic changes within the cells that comprise each of our organs. Keep in mind that the full scope of aging is a more complex process that scientists still don't fully understand, although breakthroughs are happening every day. These levels are all related: Our cellular age influences the age of our organs, which in turn influences our overall biological age. And here's the rub: *Research links our outlook to all levels of aging — from cells to organs to the whole person.* What's more, we see these connections across all age groups, from children to older adults.

In addition to my own work showing that optimists have fewer heart attacks and live longer — and that cynical women die sooner — other researchers have found that a high degree of anger also predicts early heart disease. Many of these studies, including mine, have been able to observe people for five to ten or more years, while others, such as *The Longevity Project: Surprising Discoveries for Health and Long Life from the Landmark Eight-Decade Study,* coauthored by Drs. Howard Friedman and Leslie Martin, followed people from early childhood over their lifetime. The most exciting finding of that study was that conscientious kids, defined as those who are dependable and goal oriented, live longer than kids who are less conscientious, corroborating similar results from other populations.

Outlook is even associated with preclinical

changes in our cardiovascular system, meaning changes that are evident on testing even before we have symptoms or a major clinical event, such as a heart attack. One of my colleagues and mentors, Dr. Karen Matthews, Distinguished Professor of Psychiatry at the University of Pittsburgh, has helped shape our current understanding of how aspects of outlook, including cynical hostility, influence our risk of cardiovascular disease in adulthood, even while we are still relatively young adults. For example, in one large study of healthy men and women who were between eighteen and thirty years old when they joined, Dr. Matthews and other researchers found that people with a high degree of cynical hostility had greater coronary artery calcification, a sign of atherosclerosis — pathological narrowing of blood vessels — and a harbinger of risk for future heart attack. In a related study, young adults with a higher degree of cynical hostility were more likely than less hostile people to develop high blood pressure in the first place, indicating that unwanted cardiovascular changes were happening earlier in their bodies.

Facets of outlook also predict the development of other major physical and mental health conditions, including dementia. I worked with Dr. Ben Chapman, Dr. Paul Duberstein, and colleagues to show that older adults who are highly conscientious are less likely to develop memory problems and dementia as they age, while neurotic individuals — those who have high levels of emotional distress — are more likely than their less neurotic counterparts to suffer dementia. To look more closely at outlook and brain health, I am currently leading a study (forthcoming this year) analyzing the brains of more than fourteen hundred postmenopausal women who have undergone structural magnetic resonance imaging (MRI). Because optimists tend to have healthier physical and mental health profiles, we expect to find that they will have larger frontal gray matter than the pessimists. Generally speaking, greater brain volume in this region means more neurons and better connections between them, all supporting higher capacity to think and make decisions of all sorts, termed *executive function.* We expect similar findings among women with lower cynical hostility (i.e., less anger and mistrust), as compared to those with higher cynical hostility. This research begs the question: Can you think and feel yourself younger? Obviously it's not that clear-cut, but perhaps the real fountain of youth emanates not from a cosmetic counter but from what's between your ears. The name of the game in aging is to retain as much executive function as possible for as long as possible, so that we can more fully enjoy the things that we love to do, which will keep us happier and healthier.

Evidence also links outlook with other conditions associated with aging, including stroke and cancer. Independent groups of researchers have found that optimistic older individuals are less likely than pessimists to suffer a stroke. And when it comes to cancer, evidence shows that people with distress-prone personalities may not only have a higher risk of developing cancer in the first place, but once they get it, the cancer may be more likely to recur and cause death. I should underscore that the term *cancer* actually refers to a number of distinct diseases, each with its own unique behavior. In other words, breast cancer, colon cancer, and lung cancer differ by a lot more than their location in the body, and future research needs to parse out how outlook affects different types of cancer.

In addition to these major physical illnesses, our outlook tends to steer us toward — or away from — mental health problems, even in childhood. People who score as more optimistic are less likely than pessimists to become depressed, and this holds true for high-schoolers and senior citizens alike, even when slightly different variations of optimism are assessed.

Teenagers with an optimistic explanatory style — which is related to the definition of optimism I introduced previously — are less likely than pessimistic kids to smoke cigarettes and marijuana, and less likely to exhibit antisocial behavior, such as getting into physical fights, running away from home, or being suspended from school. Grade-school-age kids who tend toward high degrees of hostility are more likely to start smoking in middle school. Even more intriguing, our outlook influences our long-term health trajectory. Personality psychologist Dr. Sarah Hampson and colleagues studied more than a thousand men and women in the Hawaii Personality and Health cohort and discovered that those who had been recognized by their preschool teachers as being conscientious, agreeable, or intellectually curious (terms that I'll define in greater detail below) grew up to be healthier forty- and fifty-year-olds, and this better health was in part due to lower rates of smoking, better eating habits, and higher educational attainment.

And what about the third level of aging, the changes that take place in our cells as they grow older? Increasingly, research is also linking our outlook to these changes of cellular aging, called "cellular senescence." Take telomeres, the specialized ends on our chromosomes (DNA) — sort of like the protective plastic on the end of shoelaces — that are vital to DNA replication. In humans, telomeres shorten with aging. Each time our cells divide and our replicates, our telomeres shorten. Enzymes in the nucleus of the cell, called telomerases, rebuild the telomeres after each shortening, but they do so incompletely. Once a cell's telomeres become too short, the DNA is highly unstable, which can result in cancerous transformation. In fact, risk of a first cancer and cancer-related death are highest among people who have the shortest telomeres. In this stage, with short telomeres, the cell can no longer replicate, and often becomes senescent, or old. And *our outlook plays a role in all of this:* Research has shown that pessimistic people have shorter telomeres. I am currently leading one of the largest studies to date on pessimism, cynicism, and telomere length in postmenopausal women in order to confirm and extend these results, which are expected within the next year.

Telomeres are not the only structures that change as cells age. Senescent cells also produce proteins called inflammatory markers, which are sort of like signal flares that cells fire off to each other during a general state of red alert. Short periods of red alert can help the body mobilize the immune system to combat a brief problem, such as an infection or wound, but when chronically activated, this inflammation wreaks havoc in the body. Inflammatory molecules such as C-reactive protein (CRP), interleukin-6 (IL-6), tumor necrosis factor-alpha (TNF-α), and intercellular adhesion molecule–1 (ICAM-1), among others, are now understood to be part of a biological pathway common to many chronic diseases including heart disease, diabetes, and cancer. There is now even a word for the link between inflammation and aging: *inflammaging*. (Incidentally, smoking markedly increases your inflammatory markers, a process that is thought to explain in part why smokers die an average of thirteen years earlier than nonsmokers. Yet another reason to put out that cigarette!) So what does inflammation have to do with outlook? Similar to the case with shorter telomeres, research shows that pessimism is associated with greater inflammation.

Shortened telomeres and increased inflammation are hallmarks of cellular aging, a.k.a. senescence, not only in white blood cells but also in other cells all over the body, including those that make up your muscles, adipose (fat) tissue, brain, kidneys, liver — you name it. Most people have never even heard of senescent cells, let alone thought about how they may be relevant to aging. It is only in the past couple of years that scientists have come to understand that *senescent cells are at the root of aging,* and that removing those cells literally stops the clock — at least if you are a mouse. In a 2011 landmark *Nature* article, Mayo Clinic scientist Dr. Darren Baker and colleagues chemically removed the senescent cells from the bodies of adult mice, who remained visibly younger during the study than the group of control mice, who carried on with all of their senescent cells and became stooped, slow, and weak. So much for growing old gracefully.

What's more, aging-associated changes in the control mice were more than skin deep: The muscle, fat, kidney, and brain tissue of the control mice showed telltale signs of aging, such as atrophy from withering and death of cells. In contrast, the cells of the experimental mice retained their youthful architecture. Furthermore, in older mice who had already started to show signs of aging, the experiment actually reversed some of these age-related changes, although more research is needed to understand just how much is reversible.

Before you race out to the nearest hospital or clinic to get the senescent cells sucked out of your body (I suspect you're thinking this, because for an instant I was, too), I should point out that this technology is not yet ready for humans, and that it will likely be years before it is. Until then, what can we do to manage the ever-gushing river of time? The good news is . . . lots of things! It is critical that we harness our outlook — this invaluable tool we were all born with, which continues to grow with us, and which is central to our health and aging — and make it work to our advantage.

OUTLOOK MAY BE THE EARLIEST AND MOST OVERLOOKED "RISK FACTOR" FOR AGING

We — meaning people in general, but also the larger medical and scientific community — may understand that there is some relationship between outlook and physical health. What we may not fully realize, however, is just how intimately tied our

27

outlook is to our own health and aging over the course of our lives, from our humblest beginnings as babies to the adults we are today, to the older people we'll become tomorrow. Our individualized patterns of thinking and feeling, some of which can be recognized as early as preschool, both precede and predict our risk of heart attack, stroke, and cancer: the number one, two, and four causes of death among U.S. adults according to the latest CDC report. What's more, attitudinal traits predict the very risk factors that are known to cause these major illnesses of aging — risk factors such as smoking, obesity, high blood pressure and cholesterol, and diabetes. *Considered in this light, our outlook may be our earliest "risk factor" for accelerated aging — before all the other traditional risk factors such as smoking and cholesterol levels that we've come to know and fear.* Each one of these traditional risk factors has the potential to rob us of a little — or a lot — of our youth. Having more than one, especially if they remain untreated, can significantly interfere with our enjoyment of adulthood and even shorten our lives. Couple that with an unhealthy outlook and we may be facing a mountain of risk. But there is an *up*side here: A great deal of aging is actually modifiable, meaning that we as individuals can do something about it. We are not entirely pawns of fate. We *do* have at least some say in the rate at which our body ages.

HOW OUR OUTLOOK GETS UNDER OUR SKIN

So how is it that our outlook can prevent and delay deeper frown lines, depression, diabetes, heart disease, and other illness? Our outlook affects our physiology in a number of ways.

We Metabolize the World One Situation at a Time

Our outlook, which colors our reaction to everything, can set in motion a physiologic chain reaction that we may not even be aware of, a process that ebbs and flows constantly. In medical terminology, this process is called the "neuroendocrine response to stress," where stress is essentially any stimulus that engages us. Our reaction to any given event, such as the intoxicating excitement of love at first sight or the wave of discomfort that wells up during a tough meeting with the boss, is reflected in our physiology. Famed scientists including Dr. Candace Pert, author of *Molecules of Emotion: Why You Feel the Way You Feel,* and

Dr. Bruce McEwen, coauthor of *The End of Stress as We Know It* and *The Hostage Brain,* have brought this message straight out of the lab and described to us in everyday terms how our thoughts and feelings affect our bodies. Our pulse quickens. Our adrenaline surges. Hormones such as cortisol and oxytocin may be released. In the case of the dreaded meeting with the boss, our body may be responding as if it is under threat. Those "threat response" systems are absolutely critical for some situations, and when activated sparingly, they can promote survival by readying us for action. In the next chapter I'll tell you about my own brush with a pride of lionesses — on foot — during which that system kicked in in a major way.

But chronic activation, like an iPod stuck on repeat, is unhealthy. The unrelenting experience of threat, whether actual or perceived, literally translates into wear and tear on body tissues, from our endothelium (the lining of our heart and blood vessels) to the neurons in our brains, to our DNA. In turn, our physiology may influence our thoughts and feelings, like traffic on a two-way street. For example, extreme fatigue, intense pain, hunger, or too-low blood pressure can make you feel tired and, understandably, down-trodden, so your thoughts in these physiologic states may tend toward the negative. Gaining more control over this traffic by flashing a mental stop sign when you start to feel anxious or giving the green light to relaxation is one key step toward living healthier, and perhaps, when practiced over time, even slowing down the aging process.

To round out this discussion, it bears mentioning that our acute responses to stress do not always promote survival. This is important, because we tend to think of acute stress responses as good and chronic, repetitive stress responses as bad. Medically, we see three distinct conditions in which the heart bears the brunt of the mind's ire during fight-or-flight arousal. The first, *mental stress-induced myocardial ischemia,* is a phenomenon in which anger, fear, and other strong (typically negative) emotions cause low blood flow to the heart muscle. The second, *takotsubo cardiomyopathy,* is also called stress cardiomyopathy or "broken-heart syndrome." In takotsubo cardiomyopathy, the heart muscle is stunned. This condition occurs following intense emotional experiences during which the apex of the heart is temporarily paralyzed by stress hormones including adrenaline and noradrenaline and unable to pump normally, causing it to resemble a takotsubo, or Japanese octopus trap. (Interestingly, myocardial stunning can also be caused by intense *positive* emotional experience, although this is rare.) Finally, strong emotions can also cause abnormalities in the heart's electrical system and precipitate arrhythmias, or abnormal heartbeats. The heart is not the only organ that can be damaged during acute stress, but it is the most noticeably affected. How we manage our responses to the world influences our health, both in the short and long term.

Our Outlook Drives Our Behaviors

The most obvious way in which outlook has an effect on our health and aging is that our attitudes are in the driver's seat when it comes to our behavior — and I'm clearly not talking about sitting quietly in the classroom with your hands folded in your lap like a good little girl or boy. Behavior encompasses almost anything you do or don't do, and is a huge player when it comes to healthy aging. If you're pessimistic about your own ability to overcome a challenge, for example, like starting an exercise program or losing weight, then you may be less likely to come up with a plan of attack, stick to that plan, and seek out medical and moral support. As I noted earlier, kids with an optimistic thinking style (which, like optimistic explanatory style, is similar to dispositional optimism) tend to steer clear of smoking and other substance use and integrate better socially, while pessimistic kids, and those with a high degree of anger, tend to have the opposite profiles. As kids grow up, their early experiences — colored by attitudes, which in turn drive behaviors — tend to snowball, such that they are able to build on prior successes, or not. Hindered by varying degrees of hopelessness or help-lessness, many are not able to reach their full potential as adults. Henry Ford summed it up best when he said, "Whether you think you can or you can't, you're right."

Outlook and Compliance with "Doctor's Orders"

Following the proverbial doctor's orders, termed *adherence* or *compliance* in medical lingo, is one of the most important things you can do for yourself as you age, and people with certain attitudes tend to do it best. Adherence is a little different from what I discussed above for health behaviors, although they are closely related. For ex-ample, people who start smoking as kids or

33

young adults will be more likely to quit smoking later in life if they adopt a plan of attack — such as setting a quit date, joining a formal smoking cessation class, and using a nicotine patch or other proven medication — and *adhere* to it. So adherence involves formulating and recognizing a plan of action and sticking to it, regardless of whether we are talking about quitting smoking, continuing an exercise program, or taking medication for blood pressure, blood sugar, or blood cholesterol. The point is that even if you've stumbled into some pitfalls in the past, hewing to a sound plan *right now* can make a huge difference for your health and aging in the present and in the future. In one study, older female optimists were more likely to stick to the dietary plan that had been recommended for them.

CARDIOVASCULAR DISEASE RISK: THE 99% AND THE 1%

Chances are you are in the camp of the 99 percent when it comes to risk of heart disease, meaning you have at least one risk factor. To understand this situation better, and to see how outlook plays a major role in why you're in the 99 percent, let's take a look at some real data on coronary heart disease (CHD), the number one killer of

American men and women and a major cause of adult death around the world. While CHD typically affects us after fifty (the age at which heart attack risk rises precipitously), the biological processes that result in heart attacks actually begin in childhood or even earlier. Autopsy studies, one of which I worked on at the Cook County morgue as an undergraduate student, show that unfortunate teens who died from accidents, suicide, or homicide already had fatty streaks and other early signs of atherosclerosis in their major arteries. As a disease, CHD is intriguing for another reason: It is almost entirely preventable through lifestyle and simple medications.

In 2010 the American Heart Association (AHA) introduced the concept of "ideal cardiac health" to guide people to live healthier and avoid cardiovascular disease (CVD, encompassing CHD, stroke, and peripheral vascular disease, or blockages in the blood vessels of the body that occur somewhere besides the heart and brain). To achieve ideal cardiac health, a person needs to avoid most of seven major risk factors known to cause and/or accelerate CVD: smoking, impaired fasting glucose (a.k.a. diabetes), high cholesterol, high blood pressure, being sedentary, eating an unhealthy diet, and being obese (with a body mass index of 30 or higher). The AHA refers to these as the "Simple 7." As you can see, all of these metrics are *modifiable,* meaning that you can do something about them. Furthermore, they do not require you to understand rocket science (homage to Ed Yong, science writer extraordinaire and creator of the Not Exactly Rocket Science blog at *Discover* magazine), spend loads of money, or adopt a complicated lifestyle. The instructions are: *Don't start smoking, and if you do, quit. Control your blood sugar, your blood cholesterol, and your blood pressure. Exercise on most days of the week. Eat reasonable portions of healthy foods, cut back on unhealthy ones, and maintain a weight that is healthy for your height.* An important aspect of ideal cardiac health is that it not only necessitates that we avoid risky behaviors (e.g., smoking), but also that we embrace positive behaviors (physical activity, healthy diet, taking steps to control blood pressure, etc). Back in the 1990s, two decades before the AHA coined the term *ideal cardiac health,* my medicine professors referred to it as "bread and butter" primary care, recognizing even then that it was a road map to preventing disease.

For people with ideal cardiac health, their

youthfulness at any age is marked by the distinct absence of CVD. To put a number on it, almost no one with ideal cardiac health has a heart attack or stroke during his or her life span. Conversely, those who rack up even four of the seven risk factors (the obese smoker with uncontrolled high blood pressure and cholesterol) face a nearly 50 percent chance of having a heart attack or stroke. Now here is the kicker: Looking across the nation, how many people do you think meet the standards for ideal cardiac health? Shockingly, less than 1 percent of American adults. So what gives? Why is something that seems so simple and is almost a guaranteed get-out-of-jail-free card for CVD so difficult to attain, and rejected by up to 99 percent of our population?

It's a question I asked myself for years as a practicing physician, and in 1999, I had a lightbulb moment. During my first year in full-time primary care practice, I began to see firsthand in my patients the living, breathing "face" of these distressing numbers. After residency training in Chicago my husband and I took our first professional positions in a large, well-established HMO practice in southern Washington state, where patients had been coming with their families since the time of the WWII ship-yards. In this semirural area, many of my patients smoked, were obese, drank alcohol to excess or were addicted to painkillers, and had symptoms of depression and anxiety. Although I had taken care of my own clinic patients during residency training, the focus had been on extremely ill, hospitalized patients, many of whom were comatose and on ventilators (respirators), or otherwise too sick to have extended conversations. So it was not until I had the benefit of seeing large numbers of the same people month after month that I began to see their common need for behavior change, as well as the widespread inertia that I learned to recognize as an immense barrier to healthy aging. One night I came home, plopped myself and my briefcase down at the dining room table, and uttered two words to my husband: "Behavior change."

"What?" he asked, opening a beer.

"Behavior change," I said, exhausted. "Almost every one of these people needs to make some major change in their *behavior* to get healthy."

He knew exactly what I was talking about, because his clinic, only three miles down the road, told the same story, as did every other physician's clinic in our large community practice. Roughly a third of my patients needed to quit smoking. Another third needed to lose twenty-five or more pounds. Yet another third had undertreated depression or anxiety. Many described toxic social and family relationships, loneliness, and outright isolation. At that time, I could think of only one person in my clinic whose fate had been sealed by genetics. She had Huntington's disease, an inherited condition involving the progressive loss of motor control and early death. Ironically, she was one of the few people who proactively sought my help to quit smoking, and she was successful. It was clear to me that for most people, their behavior, rather than genetic conditions or accidental injuries, was at the root of the medical problems responsible for their premature disability and disease.

But there was something else that I noticed as I continued to practice. Most people seemed surprisingly inert when it came to taking charge of their own health, even as they started to experience some of the harsh consequences of what they all-too-casually passed off as "normal aging." In many cases these consequences — high blood pressure, high blood sugar, feeling tired all the time — were not solely a consequence of becoming chronologically older. And yet there were a few people who took what has now become the AHA blueprint for healthy cardiovascular aging and followed the instructions as if they were commandments. What was it, I wondered, that incited those few people to adopt and maintain healthy behaviors, while the vast majority resisted, even in the face of imminent suffering and early death? Where did their volition come from?

I was so fueled by this question that I left my primary care practice and moved with my husband, baby daughter, and adopted Rottweiler three thousand miles across the country to join a three-year fellowship training program at Harvard Medical School, where I learned to design clinical trials and other types of studies in hopes of generating some answers. A decade and a half later, my career continues to organize itself around my fascination with volition, behavior, and behavior change. The surface answer, and one I've heard tossed around in medical faculty rooms for years, is that it's a simple equation of incentives — pizza tastes good *now,* cigarettes make you feel good *now,* and you can't taste, smell, or feel the benefit of a healthy heart at some distant point in the future.

Given that humans are hardwired to overvalue rewards *now* and undervalue rewards *later,* this answer seems understandable and satisfying, until one thinks about that elusive 1 percent of people — those who achieve ideal cardiac health, or even the 19 percent who get a little more than halfway there, with predictably fantastic health results. How do they do it? What motivates them? Are they pushing themselves forward toward a specific goal (looking and feeling great), pushing themselves away from an undesirable result (becoming a cardiac cripple), or both? What is the script going on inside their heads, if there is one? Are they able to defy the typical human tendency to overvalue the *now* (the brownie) and somehow turn their full attention to a future that offers favorable odds of healthy aging because they engage that future as strongly as if they could experience it *now,* almost as if they could increase the immediacy of the reward? Many of these questions go beyond what the existing research has answered, but I'll consider them further from my own perspective as a doctor and as a patient.

I believe that a big part of the mystery of the 1 percent is in our outlook — whether we can envision a positive outcome and muster the confidence and drive to work toward it, taking stock in our own abilities, our friends, and family to help us through. Earlier, I told you about the large study I led that found that optimists had more favorable cardiovascular risk profiles than pessimists. In that study, my colleagues and I looked at five of the "Simple 7," and we found that across the board, optimists had better cardiovascular risk profiles than pessimists. Now, Dr. Randi Foraker and I are leading a study to examine how optimists and pessimists measure up for all seven components of ideal cardiac health.

I am also working with Ana Progovac, a graduate student, to study something else of great interest: whether optimists and pessimists diverge on health behaviors over time. We have already found that optimists were less likely than pessimists to be smoking at the beginning of the study. The next step is to determine whether the optimistic smokers are more likely to *quit* smoking over time. We will further be able to see how cynical hostility — that deep mistrust of others — influences a person's likelihood of quitting smoking. This research will join the body of literature demonstrating that facets of our outlook do influence our ability to change behavior. For example, in the Whitehall II study of British civil servants, people with high trait anger not only started out heavier than less angry people, but over about twenty years, they also tended to gain more weight as time went by. Many more studies show that aspects of our outlook influence our behaviors over time. The implications? A healthier outlook may be like the wind in your sails when it comes to caring for your body — speeding you along on a healthier course.

Thus, our outlook affects our health and aging both directly and indirectly in myriad ways. That said, it's critical to understand that many factors — some within our control, others not — play into how quickly we become ill or age. Based on current research, we can't congratulate the optimist for steering clear of a heart attack any more than we can blame the pessimist for having one. The main point is to recognize that our outlook can be one of our strongest allies in the aging process.

Origins of Outlook
So what determines whether we look "up" or "down"? Experts estimate that about one-quarter to one-half of our outlook can be considered genetic. But the rest is a product of our life experiences, especially

those in childhood and young adulthood. If a child is born into a chaotic home life and encounters misfortune every day for years, that child may grow to expect only hardship from the world, especially if she does not acquire adequate coping skills. This is not to downplay hardship by suggesting that everything should be fine and dandy if only people could cope properly. Rather, we all know that the equation is not quite as simple as *what* one experiences — it's also *how* one experiences any given situation. Similarly, people who experience prejudice of any kind, whether motivated by race, ethnicity, gender, income, education, or some other category, may be less likely to trust others and more likely to view them as unsafe. Interestingly, not everyone who has learned from the school of hard knocks grows up to be a pessimist or a cynic, and not everyone accustomed to tasting success is an optimist. No one knows the precise origins of outlook, but we scientists are trying to unearth some of the genetic roots.

OUTLOOK GPS: GAUGING OUR ATTITUDE LATITUDE

Because our outlook is integral to aging, you may want to learn to accurately ID your traits and figure out where you fall on the landscape. It might help to think of outlook address as coordinates on a globe — attitude latitude, if you will — yielding a position we occupy on the map of the outlook world. Outlook doesn't exist on a black-and-white spectrum. Rather, it is multidimensional, produced by the intersection of a number of traits that localize each one of us at a set of unique coordinates on "planet Outlook," much like latitude, longitude, and altitude identify our physical coordinates on earth. What GPS system can we use to confirm our position and navigate this terrain? For starters, think of a few words you would use to describe yourself to a friend. We each have varying definitions for our own outlook, usually dominated by the character trait(s) with which we identify most strongly. My own strongest tendencies are hopefulness and intellectual curiosity, but I can be plagued by doubt — a combination I've dubbed "struggling optimism." Oprah espouses an unshakable "attitude of gratitude" and has positioned herself in generally positive territory, while neurotic George Costanza, from *Seinfeld,* has his feet firmly planted on an entirely different continent. Each of these "regions" on the outlook map features patterns of thinking and feeling that tend to be stable over time.

As you'll see, that doesn't mean they can't change (thank goodness!). There are several outlook regions that are recognized as potentially important for physical and mental health, and that deserve the most focus if you want to move to healthier ground. Below I discuss some of these key outlook territories.

Optimism and Pessimism

My personal favorite, optimism, is a general hopefulness for the future. Pessimism, usually considered optimism's polar opposite, is a tendency to lack hope for good things to come, or to take lack of hope one step further and expect the worst. I'll discuss optimism in greater detail in chapter 2, but for now, here is one way of thinking about it: *Optimism is the ability to see your own bright future as real, and bring it to the present.* It's as if you're able to "borrow" from your own vision — like money in the bank — to get through the hardship today, in order to make that future a reality. But instead of borrowing money, you are borrowing the psychology of success — the confidence, conviction, and other myriad furnishings of your own bright future. And unlike with a true bank account, you don't have to subtract from the total every time you make a withdrawal, because your ability to imagine is infinitely renewable. Are you thinking that this process is too hocus-pocus or something you could never get into? Take a page out of your own history: As a child, you accomplished this effortlessly in your imaginary play as you became a superhero, princess, scientist, fireman, secret agent, or whatever you foresaw for yourself. Somewhere along the way, we tend to lose sight of this built-in talent for envisioning good things and making them happen now, which is unfortunate, because this most valuable of tools doesn't cost you anything. In fact, there are significant costs associated with *not* applying hopefulness in this practical way. Afraid of disappointment, of getting your hopes up, only to have them dashed? Try the disappointment of pessimism, which can stop a person dead in her tracks toward better health.

Anger

Evolution has programmed us to experience anger, along with other emotions for which we are hardwired. Scientific knowledge aside, we all know firsthand that anger can serve the valuable purpose of alerting us to situations in which we need to take action. But as I mentioned earlier, the evidence shows that people with a high degree of anger do worse healthwise. Just as with most psychological traits, anger has several manifestations — physical aggression, verbal outbursts, pent-up rage that is more difficult to detect, and the mistrust of other people that I introduced earlier as cynical hostility. Much of my own work with outlook and aging focuses on the latter type.

The "Big Five" Personality and Character Traits

Research psychologists have sliced and diced the psyche in other ways, too. Drs. Paul Costa and Robert McCrae, at the National Institutes of Health, developed one particularly well-studied classification scheme of some of the character traits that comprise our outlook. The so-called Big Five classification refers to five broad traits that are considered to account for the majority of variation in human personality:

1. *openness to experience* — imaginative, interested in new ideas
2. *conscientiousness* — reliable, persistent, striving to achieve
3. *extroversion* — being sociable and generally positive
4. *agreeableness* — demonstrating

trust and friendliness
5. *neuroticism* — highly prone to distress

Of these five, neuroticism has been most consistently linked to negative health, and conscientiousness and openness most consistently linked to positive health. Agreeableness has not been as thoroughly studied as some of the other Big Five traits, but it does predict a person's ability to adapt in healthy ways after a disabling event. Interestingly, young adults who are less agreeable tend to be more aggressive, and to exhibit antisocial behavior.

Ikigai and Other Ineffable Qualities

In addition to the major psychological traits already described, there are aspects of our outlook that are less easily measured, but that are critical to maintaining our physical, mental, and spiritual youthfulness. They bring us joy and fulfillment, and motivate us to jump out of bed in the morning. These qualities, including compassion (which I'll discuss more in chapters 3 and 6) and sense of purpose, are more difficult to quantify in a scientific study, although there are now questionnaires to assess many of them. For some of us, such qualities may remain private, known only to our loved ones or people with whom we choose to share them. In some cases, we may not even know ourselves well enough to characterize or describe them.

Because these less tangible aspects of our outlook are more difficult to assess, research on how they affect health and aging is less available. Yet there is nothing intangible about how they affect our physical bodies. Take *ikigai* (pronounced ee-kee-guy), for example, the Japanese word for the concept of "sense of life worth living," or living life with joy and purpose. Research shows that those who affirm *ikigai* live longer than those who don't, all other things being equal. One of my goals in this book is to help you find and embrace the ineffables that are unique to you — or if you have already found them, to help you continue to espouse and augment them and encourage others to do the same.

Many of the traits I've discussed have overlapping features, but are not completely synonymous, and there are many tools that researchers use to determine our unique combination of traits. First, there are questionnaires. Coupling these questionnaires with related biological information such as blood pressure, hormone levels, EKG and

EEG (electrical heart and brainwaves), and brain imaging gets us one step closer to how aspects of our outlook affect our physiology and ultimately our health. Scientists may soon be able to see recognizable telltale neuroimaging patterns associated with each one of our traits, similar to the way in which famed neuroscientist Dr. Richard Davidson (and one of my earliest research advisers), coauthor of *The Emotional Life of Your Brain: How Its Unique Patterns Affect the Way You Think, Feel, and Live — and How You Can Change Them,* has categorized distinct neural signatures of emotional style.

BRIGHTER OUTLOOK, BETTER HEALTH SPAN

People often wonder, "Can I change my outlook?" Psychologists have posed this question as well, and have demonstrated that generally, outlook is relatively stable past age twenty or thirty, meaning that an optimist tends to remain an optimist. But we also know that our brains are *plastic,* or changeable. So what is the bottom line? As much as I've seen in clinical practice that unhealthy behavior can remain stubbornly consistent, I've also witnessed many instances in which it changes for the better. *People can change,* even if they already have chronic, often "incurable" conditions.

Victor, a middle-aged patient of mine, developed high blood pressure and high cholesterol in his fifties. Both of these conditions, which may have been hereditary given his strong family history, increased his risk of heart disease. When I met Victor, he had already been grossly overweight for many years, and he felt "as weak as an old man." But for all his complaining, he had done little to change his situation. Then, seemingly without explanation, he lost more than fifty pounds in less than a year and gained his strength and his strut back. One day, after not seeing him for several months, I walked into the exam room and did a double take, momentarily thinking I had the wrong patient. He looked amazing! He had worked out five days a week, exercised portion control, and stuck to his medication schedule. What was it that helped Victor finally see that he had a say in his own health? How did he identify the pathway to change and then manage to stay on that "yellow brick road"? His hat went off to his mother, who after hearing him talk about getting healthy for decades, finally took action and told him, "Victor, you *can* do this." She engaged other family and friends to do the same, so he heard this message many times from multiple people, and began to believe it. Once he started to see and feel results after the first few workouts, he locked on to that mental picture of success "like a bulldog on a bone," as he described it.

While what you need to do to lose weight or lower cholesterol is fairly obvious, effecting change at the cellular level to prevent cells from becoming senescent is less clear-cut and still in the nascent stages of research. Someone recently asked me, "How do I lengthen my telomeres?" It's a fair question and reflects what many of us often wonder about: "How do I keep myself as young as possible on all levels — cells, organs, the whole of me — even as time marches on?" If I told you there was a single solution, such as a pill, an exercise, a mantra, or some dietary method to stay young, telomeres and all, I'm guessing you would move heaven and earth to embrace it.

At this stage, modern medicine is not aware of any single such entity for humans. (As I described earlier, removal of senescent cells in mice *is* a veritable fountain of youth, but that technique is, at present, available only for the mice.) There is evidence that people who boost their omega-3 fatty acids by eating a diet high in fish such as salmon and tuna have lower risk of cardiovascular disease and slower telomere degradation over time, but I don't think we can go so far as to call fish oil *the* Holy Grail. Regular physical exercise may be the closest thing we have to a fountain of youth, as we'll discuss further in chapter 5, but the main problem with exercise is that so few people in the nation are doing it regularly! Some scientists have speculated and shown preliminary evidence to support that meditation and similar practices can keep telomeres healthy, perhaps by slowing the rate at which they shorten. Researchers at the University of California, San Francisco, recently published the first study linking meditation to positive psychological change, including increased sense of control, lower emotional negativity, an increased sense of purpose in life, *and* increased telomerase activity. (Recall that telomerases are the enzymes that build up the telomeres after each cellular division, to keep them long and healthy.) So while each of these and other proven steps by themselves may maintain our health, in aggregate, they set us on a path to healthier aging, including keeping those all-important telomeres as long as possible for as long as possible! By "healthier aging" I am referring to the full gamut, including physical and mental well-being and health behaviors such as (not) smoking and physical exercise. Your outlook is integral to whether you walk this path — or not.

Whatever your goals are as you age, we all know that the road to better health can be tough to walk. But people do find it and stick to it. People, like Victor, who are overweight *do* successfully exercise and shape up. People who are weighed down by depression, diabetes, and many other chronic conditions *do* get better. One of the things I love best about being a doctor is delivering the recurrent message to people that they can do great things with their health and modify aging.

If you count yourself as one of those who naturally take a more pessimistic, cynical, or neurotic view of things, don't despair. I've dedicated chapters 3, 4, and 5 to steps for changing your outlook in small but noticeable ways. Take cognitive behavioral therapy (CBT), a tried-and-true method of learning to see situations in a different light. In people with depression and anxiety, CBT has been shown to actually change the neural circuits in the brain that underlie the way we process our anxieties and fears. The brain is, in effect, wired for second chances, and you can train it to do the "bright" thing. Sometimes, no formal training at all is required. People may spontaneously change after experiencing what experts call a frame shift, a major change in the way a person views life. It may be brought on by a shocking or catastrophic event, such as the illness of a friend or family member. In my own case, bouncing back from my life-threatening heart condition in college brought all of my blessings into sharp relief: first I felt uncertainty and fear, then gratitude for my life and everything in it. Somewhere in the midst of those feelings emerged an inviolable hope. This experience inspired me to study how a person's outlook can improve her health span.

It also inspired me to communicate to others that being hopeful doesn't equate with turning one's back on reality or losing one's head in the clouds. In fact, true optimism, as strictly defined by psychologists, is closer to realism than most people recognize, and has little to do with a Sunshine Sally caricature. Having the confidence to believe that good things can and will happen and then working — sometimes really hard — toward those future goals is one of our most valuable attributes. To shun this glorious process as pie-in-the-sky or at-tempt to blunt it with excessive caution is to throw away a priceless tool for overcoming obstacles. Following our goals and desires with excitement and vigor necessitates believing on some level that they are attainable. Otherwise, why get up in the morning?

In the next chapter I'll introduce you to several "faces" of optimism, one of which is mine, to illustrate how not everyone experiences the same trait in precisely the same way. As a struggling optimist, I've been able to identify some of the key "ingredients" necessary to keep myself looking up. Despite the many successes in my own life, I often still sense a strong undercurrent of unease tugging at my ankles like an ominous under-tow, discouraging me from diving into opportunities wholeheartedly. My solution? To view skepticism and hopelessness in the same way I view physical ailments: They need tending to. As a physician I am inti-mately acquainted with the physical heart — those four chambers, the valves that separate them, and the arteries that feed them. But the physical organ is not the only part of a person that needs care and treat-ment.

Over the years of placing my stethoscope

on people's chests, abdomens, and blood vessels, I have heard sounds of hopefulness and resilience. But I have also listened to tones of despair, isolation, and anger. After stepping back from the obvious circumstances of disease — the sudden heart attack, the liver abscess, the smoldering path to emphysema — I learned to pay attention to the attitudes that both permeate and shape each person's unique circumstances. Now, as a forty-three-year-old physician who has walked the corridors of several major academic hospitals, I do more than pay attention to these attitudes. I try to help people cultivate healthier ones.

NATIONAL OUTLOOK

If you accept that attitudes are a driver of health, and you look at our dismal national health report card (summed up in the 2003 Institute of Medicine report, "U.S. Health in International Perspective: Shorter Lives, Poorer Health"), when it comes to cardiovascular disease, you can make the argument that what's needed to turn things around for an aging nation is a better approach to cultivating a healthy outlook. We'll discuss this topic in chapter 8. Ideally, a healthy outlook is instilled in us as children by our parents, teachers, friends, and positive experiences — or the important lessons we glean from negative experiences. Take optimism, for example. Not only does early optimism, or at the very least, absence of early pessimism, encourage problem solving, but it may also help us preserve the good health we're born into as children. Believing from a young age that you will enjoy a long and healthy life is no small thing. In one recent study, about 14 percent of the twenty thousand seventh- through twelfth-graders surveyed believed they would not live beyond age thirty-five. These kids were more likely than those who projected a longer life to go on to experience serious health outcomes and negative life events, such as fight-related injury, police arrest, or a diagnosis of HIV/AIDS as young adults. In the case of HIV/AIDS, youth who believed they would not live beyond age thirty-five were twice as likely to acquire the disease.

In a fascinating follow-up study of the teenagers over a one-year period, just over half of those who had predicted early death now predicted greater life expectancy. The two most notable factors associated with this change of heart were increased self-esteem and establishing positive social bonds with adults. (We'll discuss social support more in chapter 5.) These results should incite us to give our children explicit instruction on how to live hopefully and healthfully, ideas that are increasingly part of discussions among educational boards, scientists, and parents alike. Outlook is integral to these discussions.

On the one hand, this all seems so obvious as to go without saying. On the other hand, if we all truly understood and lived by this principle, we would uniformly seek to change our own outlook for the better and help foster a brighter one for our kids. In his book *The Optimistic Child,* distinguished researcher and author Dr. Martin Seligman relates how the late Dr. Jonas Salk coined the term *psychological immunization* to describe the process of providing kids with psychological tools, akin to antibodies, to face the vicissitudes of life. In the chapters that follow I'll bring in many colleagues of different backgrounds to lay the conceptual groundwork for future clinical trials designed to change outlook, and thereby effect healthy aging.

OUTLOOK MATTERS FOR *YOU*

The mind-body link is critical for everyone — not just children whose brains are growing rapidly, and not just for people with depression, anxiety, or other serious mental health conditions. In 2003, the late Dr. Stephen Strauss, former director of the National Center for Complementary and Alternative Medicine and world-renowned virologist, made a site visit to the division of Harvard Medical School where I was training as a research fellow in general internal and integrative medicine. After I gave a brief summary of my research interests in behavior change and quitting smoking, Dr. Strauss stared me down and remarked, "How is it that an internist is doing the work of a psychiatrist?" Without thinking, I retorted with what I had found to be true as a full-time primary care doctor: "Anyone who has ever practiced internal medicine understands that it *is* psychiatry." The room erupted into laughter and vigorous nods. "Fair enough," Dr. Strauss said, smiling. In other words, for the person who's just had a heart attack, you have to convince him that the way he thinks about his body, diet, and life needs to change — first comes the mental shift, then the behavior change. In some cases, just getting people to change their unhealthy routine can help bring on the mental shift even before they are fully aware of the positive effects of doing so. Even more challenging are the psychologi-

cal gymnastics of *preventive* health care —
convincing people who are apparently
healthy, but often deceptively so, to change
their behavior in order to avoid the heart
attack, stroke, or other problem in the first
place, by quitting smoking, controlling
cholesterol and blood pressure, exercising,
and managing mood and stress.

When I graduated from medical school,
my mother gave me my first set of business
cards. They featured the famous quote from
Voltaire "It is the charge of the physician to
amuse the patient while nature effects a
cure." The modern translation: The doctor
helps the patient maintain a healthy attitude, which in turn facilitates the body's
natural healing abilities. This book is just
that — an instruction manual to understand
and harness the power of outlook, and to
recognize that the "sweet spot" is certainly
not one-size-fits-all. Those of us who aren't
yet living in our sweet spot can choose from
a wealth of strategies to move ourselves
closer to this healthier vantage point. Main-
stream medicine has been criticized by lay-
people and health scientists alike for not
incorporating outlook into the overall health
equation, and in some cases for actively
excluding it from any discussion of health
and disease. But with all the exciting new

research and experts who are recognizing its importance, I predict that outlook will soon be more widely employed as both a preventive and therapeutic medicine. One of my career goals is to lay the scientific groundwork to give doctors and other health care providers the data not only to prescribe attitudinal change in the same way we prescribe aspirin or statin medication, but also to be able to quantify its impact on health: "Mrs. Jones, based on results from clinical trials, a healthy outlook can be expected to lower your risk of heart disease by X percent over X years." Medicine is, indeed, looking *up*.

2
THE MANY FACES
OF OPTIMISM

Smile and the world smiles with you. Turn
that frown upside down. Don't worry, be
happy. These bumper-sticker mantras are
meant to inspire an optimistic outlook, yet
for many, they trigger the opposite: eyeball
rolling, ridicule, and even anger. It's no
wonder — such blithe mentalities often
don't address the complexities and serious-
ness of life's challenges. Who wants to hear
advice to "be happy" or "hope for the best"
while facing a home foreclosure, loss of a
job, divorce, or a serious medical diagnosis?
On the one hand, it's not realistic or helpful
to simply tell people who are facing misfortune to think themselves happy, rich, and
well. Yet as we've already seen, the research
shows that regardless of your socioeconomic
or personal circumstances, outlook is important when it comes to health and longevity.
This discussion gets even more interesting
when we consider that the character trait of

optimism, just like all aspects of our outlook, doesn't cost us anything and doesn't interact with medications we may be taking. I believe that optimism can be an invaluable tool for our health and aging. Yet we not only shy away from fully utilizing it, but in some cases we actively denounce it. *Why?*

In discussions of optimism in the media, in the classroom, and around the dinner table, the terminology has become a big hurdle and confused the issue. I'm referring to the erroneous assumption that *trait* or *dispositional optimism* — the tendency to generally expect good things in the future — is the same as the *optimistic bias,* defined as the tendency to be systematically wrong, or biased, in predicting that future events will be positive. To understand the terminology better, I turned to Dr. William Klein, associate director of the Behavioral Research Program at the National Cancer Institute, who along with his colleague and optimistic bias pioneer, Dr. Neil Weinstein, has produced key research to define and distinguish these two very different concepts. The optimistic bias is also sometimes referred to as "unrealistic optimism." An extreme example of someone having an optimistic bias or being unrealistically optimistic is captured in the following statement: "I don't need to try and save any money for retirement, because everything will work out just fine." Most of us can see that such a plan is not only irresponsible; it is more than likely a recipe for disaster. When people in research studies are asked whether they are above average on a number of metrics — intelligence, wealth, education, health — more than half say yes. But since only half can be above average, you begin to see the disconnect.

Now, it may seem counterintuitive, says Dr. Klein, but actual optimists typically do not have an optimistic bias. In studies that have measured both the optimistic bias and trait optimism in the same people, the correlation between the two is very, very low (and sometimes zero), meaning that they are essentially unrelated. Optimists do tend to rate themselves above average on a number of health metrics, such as physical activity and other healthy behaviors, so they *are* comparatively optimistic. But in truth, optimists actually are above average health-wise — they exercise more, have lower rates of high blood pressure and high cholesterol, smoke less, etc. — so they are not being unrealistic or biased when they make these comparisons. Comparative optimism only spills over into unrealistic optimism or an optimistic bias when it isn't true. To use the retirement savings example, optimists simultaneously foresee a bright future and start saving for it.

The reality is that trait optimism shares very little with those bumper sticker mantras, which seem to be unrealistically optimistic. People who score as optimists on the formal research scales show themselves to be proactive, expert copers who hit problems head-on, and they are actually much closer to what many of us would refer to as "realists." So the anti-optimism schools of thought that vilify what they view as empty, harebrained optimism are in fact largely attacking the idea of encouraging people to amplify their own optimistic bias. Everyone can see how an extreme optimistic bias can be very dangerous, because it can make you careless when you really do need to be pragmatic. An extreme optimistic bias can even be detrimental to health, a classic example being the misconception held by some smokers that cigarettes are harmful to other smokers, but not to them personally.

Through the unfortunate synonymous misuse of the terms *optimism* and *optimistic bias,* many people have been led to believe that trait optimism is not only unhelpful, but it is actively harmful. Some have even gone so far as to suggest that it may be better to be slightly depressed in order to avoid the pitfalls of making overly optimistic predictions. Given the immense toll depression takes on physical health, this prescription does not make good clinical sense. Others have suggested that we need to balance our optimism with pessimism. But if that were true, then the "in-betweens" — i.e., those who score above the most pessimistic people but below the most optimistic — would have the healthiest behaviors and the fewest heart attacks and strokes, and would live the longest. But as I've already shown you, that is not what the research demonstrates. Instead, the optimists have the lowest rates of disease and death (and pessimists the highest). If we are to understand the research findings correctly and "live" the science, it is critical that we clear up these widespread misconceptions. What I'll show you is that you don't need to trade hope for realism. You can equally embrace both, and both are good for health and healthy aging.

A second reason I believe we don't fully utilize optimism as a tool for our health and aging is the misperception that we have to become "turbocharged" optimists in order to reap any associated benefits. Optimism, like most aspects of our outlook, has many faces, and you don't have to be a poster child for the stereotype. For those of you who are not yet convinced of this, it's enough for now to know that you don't have to go skipping through the woods singing "Kumbaya" to see the future as bright. In the next section I offer three examples of real, everyday people (I am one of them) who exhibit optimistic qualities in different ways. I use these examples to help you see your own face in this amazing character trait, but it's important for you to understand that they are not part of the published scales, and have not been formally identified in research studies. (They are, however, readily apparent to me from my vantage point as a clinician.) Each of us may wear one or more of these optimistic faces at some point, or we may tend toward one for most of our lives. In reality, we don't go around administering research tests and formal labels to everyone we meet, but we can glean clues about people's outlook by listening and watching. Through close observation of myself and others, I've seen many faces of optimism, each a little bit different in character, but all, in their own way, looking *up*.

THE PRAGMATIC OPTIMIST

Just as adopting a hopeful outlook doesn't mean ignoring reality or blindly walking into danger, expecting bad things to happen isn't necessarily pessimistic, especially when those situations can be effectively anticipated, managed, neutralized, and sometimes even turned into good things. In fact, in some cases, the very act of *not* expecting misfortune can almost guarantee it through sheer lack of preparedness. The most positive outcomes may result from scanning the horizon, anticipating possible scenarios, and formulating a plan B if things become unstable. Having contingency plans and solutions at the ready separates the habit of blind hope from the practice of inspired pragmatism. I saw the clearest example of this pragmatic face of optimism while on safari in sub-Saharan Africa.

In the summer of 1999, after finishing three arduous years of internal medicine residency training at the University of Chicago, my husband and I took out a cash advance on our credit card, waved good-bye to Lake Michigan, and boarded a plane for Johannesburg, South Africa. For the next two months while traveling through game parks in five countries, our primary task was to wake up each day and experience for ourselves what we had only been able to read about in *National Geographic.* We arrived in Victoria Falls, Zimbabwe, for a walking safari with one of the most experienced guides in the entire country, who had come so highly recommended from the Sierra Club's southern African representative — "Whatever you do, you *must* find Leon Varley!" — that we didn't even consider using anyone else. He displayed a relentless preparedness for the dangerous unpredictability of the natural world while maintaining an unwavering expectation that beautiful, awesome experiences would emanate from it. He ultimately expected the best in the face of uncertainty — the definition of a true optimist — but getting to that point involved an expectation of what could go wrong and, most important, a plan for overcoming those barriers.

"Mista Vah-ley," as his name was pronounced by the native Zimbabwean Ndebele staff, was a veteran sportsman and tracker who had been leading ecotourist walking safaris for decades. His motto was, "If you're not going to walk it, stay at home and watch it on TV." Early on the morning of our expedition, Leon came to collect us at our hotel. After introducing us to the other passengers, he motioned a command

71

to the trackers, Stephen and Obert, who quickly loaded us into the trucks to begin our seven-hour, mostly off-road trek to Chizarira National Park, one of Zimbabwe's most remote locations.

By our third tire change, we were dusted from head to toe with a hot, turmeric-colored powder from the ancient elephant trails locals used as roads. Finally we arrived at our first camp. Without a moment's hesitation Leon gathered everyone and launched into the Safety Talk. His voice was clear and calm but stern. "Over the next week you must listen and you must follow directions at all times. And there is one thing that you must not do, unless I tell you to do it. If we are confronted by lions, *you must not run.*"

He went on to explain how most charges from animals in the bush were false. "Ninety-five percent of the time, the animal will stop when it realizes that you are not prey. This is why you must not run. The only time you will run is if I tell you to run. If I tell you to run to the left, you must run to the left." He gestured very deliberately with his strong, tanned arm cocked at ninety degrees, as if he were directing an airplane. Then he turned to the other half of our semicircle and gestured in the opposite direction. "If I tell you to run to the right, you must run to the right." He ended with a definitive reassurance. "No matter what happens, I have a plan. At fifty meters the gun goes up. At twenty-five meters I drop the animal." I absorbed these instructions, half-bemused and half-terrified. In my then-naïveté, Leon seemed to me like a caricature, and I even speculated he might be putting on the drill-sergeant airs to heighten everyone's experience.

Over the next week, we traversed half of the elephant trails in Chizarira and spotted a breathtaking array of wildlife: a running pack of wild dogs, a leopard perched in a tree, a herd of elephants standing in a dry riverbed methodically swinging their trunks from side to side, divining the flow of unseen water beneath the arid ground. But the trackers looked about restlessly, dissatisfied that we had not yet seen a lion. Leon revered lions above all other "big five" animals — the other four being elephant, buffalo, rhino, and leopard, so designated because they have long been considered the most difficult to track on foot — and was determined to find them. On the morning of the seventh day, as Leon drove our vehicle in search of more game, Obert suddenly yelled, leaped out, and pointed to a long, jagged line in the sand. "That was made by a zebra's hoof," Leon explained. "The zebra was dragged across the road a few hours ago by a lioness. We are going to pursue them."

By this time we all knew the drill: Obert led our single-file line, waving his stick over the ground to expose snakes. Leon walked second, resting his rifle on his shoulders. Stephen brought up the rear, and the rest of us marched dutifully in between. We continued on for about two hours, when suddenly we heard a low, deep grunt. From Leon's storytelling at our nightly campfires, I recognized the sound as the warning call of a lioness. As we burst into a clearing, we surprised the entire pride. Leon bellowed, "There they are!" as several of them sprung to their feet and charged us while the others turned and disappeared into the foliage. Leon and Obert were shouting, waving their arms, and raising their guns up and down. As the lionesses came at us I was overwhelmed with the primal compulsion to run for my life — my fight-or-flight signal was on Mach 10. I started to turn but then heard Leon shouting, "DO NOT RUN. DO NOT RUN!" There was no time to think or plan. Everyone desperately grabbed on to everyone else. Mindlessly clenching the arms and shoulders of the people on either side of me, I planted my feet and held my ground. But the man in front of me — Jim, a middle-aged attorney from Texas — turned around and started to run. Several of us reached out to tether him, shrieking until he finally stopped in his tracks.

Within less than a minute (that seemed like an hour), the approaching lionesses halted and made a hasty retreat. We never saw or heard them again. Everyone staggered to catch their breath while the trackers surveyed the footprints, both leonine and human. Obert soon saw the evidence of Jim's wayward footprints and looked up at him, mocking a finger-shake. All of us, including Jim, burst into uncontrollable laughter. "I guess that Safety Talk was pretty important, Leon," I uttered, holding on to my aching belly muscles. Leon was unfazed. He sauntered among us, clearly pleased with this interactive sighting. In a lifetime of leading walking safaris, he had only ever had to "drop" one animal.

His approach was the best example I'd seen yet of expecting the best in the midst of life's roaring uncertainty: He anticipated danger and adapted to tough situations. But his meticulous attention to detail and level of forethought did not subdue his great expectations — he was never guardedly optimistic. Rather, he wholeheartedly hoped for the best, formulated levelheaded plans, and took action to execute them. He was my new hero.

THE INCREMENTAL OPTIMIST

On a scale of one to ten, Leon undoubtedly would have scored as a picture-perfect optimist. I didn't administer any question-naires to him while we were exploring the bush, as my skills of perception were other-wise engaged in trying to stay alive. But not everybody starts out like Leon — some people have to build optimism one step at a time. Helen, a patient of mine, had several lions in the clearing, if you will. She was able to face these beasts one at a time over several years, building her skills bit by bit as she gained the experience and confidence to change her life. To illustrate this process, I've termed her an *incremental* optimist.

Helen, a vibrant professional woman in her sixties, was a clinic patient of mine while I was in Boston for research training. From one perspective, she had everything going for her. The manager of a large nonprofit organization and the wife of a respected and successful executive, she led what seemed like a great life. She and her husband made plenty of money, had two grown children, and several beautiful grandchildren. Helen exercised daily, traveled often, and spent lots of time with family and friends at their house on Cape Cod. She always showed up to my clinic in stunning clothes, with a hairstyle as hip as the leather pumps accentuating her toned calves.

But Helen had several silent hazards on her trail — silent in the sense that they hadn't yet resulted in catastrophic health problems. She was "apparently healthy," a phrase acknowledging that people can be medical icebergs, with potential disaster lurking beneath an ostensibly sound exterior. The first problem was her pack-a-day cigarette habit of several decades. The second was her weight. Despite her vigorous exercise schedule, she had a body mass index (BMI) of 26, putting her in the "overweight" category. Driving some of this excess weight was her alcohol intake — three to four glasses of wine a night, her third hazard. (People tend to underreport the amount of alcohol they drink, so her true consumption may have been higher.) While many people don't consider three to four drinks per day to be excessive, it actually is well over the recommended limit for women of one drink per day, and is considered hazardous because it is associated with increased risk of medical problems, interpersonal problems, and accidents. The fourth hazard was the fact that her husband, who also drank to excess, was verbally abusive and controlling. He dined very late in the evening, often hours after Helen, and insisted that she clean up the dinner dishes that same night, even if it meant scrubbing them in the wee hours of the morning when she was already exhausted.

The fifth and by far the biggest hazard was the fact that Helen did not appear to recognize how dangerous the other four conditions were to her health. I thought at first she didn't truly understand the risks, or just didn't want to acknowledge them. But as I got to know her better, I realized she was feeling overwhelmed at having so much to change healthwise. Even using a treadmill five times a week was not enough to cancel out the negative effects of smoking, overconsumption of alcohol, and her emotionally toxic home life. Paralyzed by indecision, she didn't know where to start.

Let me illustrate Helen's case with some concrete numbers from published data on the lifetime risks of cardiovascular disease. Women around Helen's age who have two or more major cardiovascular disease risk factors have about a one in three chance of dying of a heart attack or stroke by age eighty. Now compare that with the risk of women with only one major cardiovascular risk factor (roughly one in four chance) and with women whose risk is considered ideal, either because they don't have any risk factors or they are expertly managing the risk factors that they do have (roughly one in ten chance). As you can see, this stuff really matters for your health span and your life span! And these trends pertain to men as well.

After I had taken Helen's medical and social history and performed her physical exam, I ordered some basic blood work and told her I wanted to see her in two to four weeks to review her lab work and tackle some of these issues. I suggested that we begin with the smoking, pointing out her own temporary past success with quitting smoking. Even brief periods of quitting are a major predictor of future success, and should be acknowledged. She nodded, but then turned away. "I'm just not sure I'm ready. I don't know if I can do it again." Helen was clearly suffering from a crisis in confidence, and a pessimism that wouldn't allow her to envision herself changing and succeeding at any one of these obstacles. I decided to let it go for now and planned to bring it up again on the next visit.

Helen surprised me a few weeks later when she strutted into my office and announced that she wanted to try to quit smoking. "I remember myself before I smoked — and when I quit," she told me. "And I can see myself that way again." She was unwittingly using a motivational interviewing technique called *looking back,* a tool clinicians use to help people change all kinds of behaviors, including smoking. Looking back helps people remember their own success in the past in order to increase their motivation and confidence to act now. The way I like to think about looking back is that you're essentially borrowing optimism from the past. Later on we'll get into its counterpart, *looking forward,* which involves envisioning oneself as already changed — i.e., having already quit smoking, having already attained a healthy body weight, etc.

In her thirties and again in her forties, Helen had been able to quit smoking for more than a year on several occasions. I pulled out a calendar and she chose her quit date while I wrote out a prescription for medication to help her. We reviewed the high-risk situations — arguments with her family or her husband, being short-staffed at work, feeling frustrated or low, and other situations in which she anticipated being tempted to smoke — and came up with a plan of action for each one. Optimistic pragmatism at work!

When we spoke briefly by phone on her quit day, she sounded pretty stressed. Yet a month later, Helen showed up to clinic as a nonsmoker. (Spoiler alert: I recently took her to lunch to celebrate more than five years of being smoke-free.) At the time, having this new success under her belt had bolstered her belief and hope that she could achieve her goal of long-term abstinence through preparedness, flexibility, persistence, and hard work. That month was no cakewalk, as any former smoker knows. Her success allowed us to begin talking about cutting down her wine intake — a discussion that we continued for the next couple of years, coming up with different strategies at each office visit.

By this point, Helen's liver function (blood test) results were abnormal. Additional tests pointed to a diagnosis of steatohepatitis, also called "fatty liver," caused by the alcohol. These abnormal lab results not only provided concrete proof that the drinking was harming her but also fueled her motivation to continue cutting down: As Helen watched her test results improve every few months, she knew it was because of her own actions. Then somewhere along the way she had the idea — and subsequently developed the volition — to schedule her exercise during the evenings, when she typically sat in the living room and drank wine with her husband. Consequently, she was up walking or biking instead of sitting inside drinking and eating empty calories.

In the course of a year she lost about twenty pounds, putting her BMI back in the healthy range. "I'm actually making progress," she said, beaming, one day while we reviewed her measurements and labs. I could see that Helen was gaining confidence about her own ability to achieve these health-related milestones. Although two glasses of wine — beginning at dinnertime and extending into couch time afterward — was a major improvement from her previous alcohol intake, this was still twice the maximum daily recommendation for women, putting her at higher risk of breast cancer and other health problems. (It's important to note that we still need more research in this area in order to fine-tune warnings about moderate alcohol intake, because people metabolize alcohol at different rates depending on their genetic makeup, which may in turn modify their risk for conditions such as breast cancer.) Further, the two nightly glasses of wine were making her feel sluggish, and she had a harder time waking up the next morning. Despite her desire to cut down further, Helen confessed that she had hit a wall — but I couldn't quite figure out why.

Her husband's drinking had escalated and he was becoming increasingly erratic. In a drunken state the previous year, he had even haphazardly thrown a wineglass in her direction. Throughout their marriage she had known that he had a problem with alcohol, leading to abusiveness, but she had never felt like she was in a position to do much about it. They had both grown up in an era when the man was the breadwinner whose wishes ruled the day, and that was that. Even when Helen had become successful with her own career, and brought home considerable bacon, these roles failed to change, essentially trapping her in a split life: She ran the show at work but returned home each evening subservient. She needed more than a few office visits to devise a safe passage out of this situation.

Trying to inch her way up, Helen was like

an amateur rock climber attempting to scale what to her felt like El Capitan, and she needed help at each step to manage a foothold here (quit smoking) and a stable handhold there (cut down on drinking and lose weight). Through a combination of her own drive and my help, she had been able to ascend to a certain point, but now she was stuck partway up the cliff — she couldn't confront her controlling husband or cut down to a safer level of drinking — and was unable to chart a path to the top. I knew the person to get her going again was Ben, a local psychologist who had successfully treated several of my other patients.

After seeing Ben for about a year and employing a number of strategies that you'll learn more about in chapter 4, Helen made the discovery of a lifetime. "I now understand that I am worth taking care of," she told me earnestly during her next visit. As an aside, optimists tend to have healthy self-esteem, but this is not universally true. With help, Helen was learning to strengthen some of her optimism "muscles," and had also made major progress in the self-esteem department. Her realization in turn catapulted her toward healthier behavior: She replaced the two nightly glasses of wine with an exercise class, supplementing her daily treadmill run. She still attends the class to this day, but now as the instructor! This increased morale bolstered her courage to speak plainly to her husband. She told him that she would not be able to continue with the current situation, and suggested AA and a counselor, both of which he agreed to. As his own health was now rapidly deteriorating, he had become more motivated to take action.

Helen's situation is an important reminder that circumstances *can* change — through a combination of a healthy outlook, strategy, hard work, and, sometimes, luck. Here's where I really want to focus your attention. If Helen had allowed a fatalistic attitude to prevail from the outset, she would still be an overweight alcohol-dependent smoker trapped in a toxic emotional relationship. As such, she was gutting her chances of healthy aging.

What's also important to underscore is that even for people who already have the risk factors — the elevated blood pressure, blood sugar, blood cholesterol, etc. — *treatment matters*! This means that if you have high blood pressure, you can really help yourself and anyone you care about by taking medication, eating healthier, exercising, and getting your blood pressure down to a normal range, typically less than 130/80 mm Hg, although 110/70 is perfect for just about all adults. Among adults who are Helen's age or older, controlling risk factors is associated with a marked reduction in risk of cardiovascular disease. The bottom line? Even if Helen had only been able to accomplish one of her goals, such as quitting smoking, she would have dramatically improved her situation. But we both knew that she had it in her to keep going, and as it happened, she managed *all* of her risk factors and dramatically lowered her chances of dying from a heart attack or stroke in the next few years. And what's more, any extra years gained were now more likely to be ones in which she enjoyed good physical and mental health, thereby compressing her morbidity and improving her health span.

Through all of this, Helen was able to do more than merely excise the medical don'ts — don't smoke, don't drink to excess, etc. These are all critical, of course, but they are only part of the equation. She also began to do the things that made her feel alive, and she no longer lived each day in fear. And what sparked the beginning of Helen's journey back to good health and sustained her along the way? Her outlook. Helen's belief that she could change, supported by various techniques and experts along the way, was as important as the prescription drugs she swallowed and the medical diagnostics that guided her treatment.

THE STRUGGLING OPTIMIST

Through hard work, support, and taking it one step at a time, Helen arrived at a place, both physically and mentally, that squarely planted her in optimistic territory, where she enjoyed much better health. However, that's not to say once you arrive there, you're a local for life. Many people who consider themselves somewhat optimistic, myself included, take frequent side trips through the valleys of pessimism and doubt, perhaps more often than we'd like. These are the struggling optimists, and while this breed generally maintains a hopeful outlook, we exert a lot of energy trying to keep ourselves on solid, hopeful ground — and not always succeeding.

Pop quiz: On a scale of 0 to 4 (0 being "I disagree a lot" and 4 being "I agree a lot"), what number would you assign to this statement when describing yourself? *"In uncertain times, I usually expect the best."* This is the first question on the Life Orientation Test, Revised (LOT-R), which I'll show you in full in chapter 3. The LOT-R is used by research psychologists to measure optimistic and pessimistic attitudes. Dr. Michael Scheier, chair of psychology at Carnegie Mellon University and a colleague of mine, created the LOT with his then-graduate student, Dr. Michael Bridges, and his career-long collaborator, Dr. Charles Carver. They intended the LOT-R to be an easy, accurate method of determining a person's expectations for the future. Their goal was to relate those expectations to health outcomes. Drs. Scheier and Carver, authors of *Perspectives on Personality,* are some of the first scientists to connect an optimistic outlook with physical health. In a 1999 study — the first of its kind — Dr. Scheier and colleagues showed that among cardiac patients who had recently undergone bypass surgery, pessimists were more likely than optimists to be readmitted to the hospital following surgery. Together, we recently replicated that finding in a second study.

The first time I read the LOT-R scale, I was a new assistant professor of medicine and it had been almost ten years since I'd met Leon Varley. I distinctly remember how that first question gave me pause. To be able to truthfully agree with that statement, a person would have to have a *lot* to bring to the table. If I had to describe my own "positive future expectation," could I honestly answer that this was true for me *most of the time*? No, I could not. But why not? I had many reasons to expect the best — I had made it through heart surgery, had found a great husband and produced two vivacious kids, and had been able to pursue my passion for biology as both a doctor and a researcher. I had even stood my ground against charging lionesses and lived to tell the tale with bliss and rapture. Yet uncertainty was everywhere. So many responsibilities, and my doubts that I could fulfill them, weighed on me in no particular order: improving the lives of my patients; trying to contribute to the world's scientific knowledge; paying bills; keeping my home presentable so that guests didn't take me for a heathen; and the "mother" of all tasks, raising my daughters to be healthy, self-sufficient, happy young ladies, while simultaneously keeping my marriage solid and my body healthy. Even though I actively worked toward these goals, on many days it felt like slogging through mud. I continued to ask myself: Why couldn't someone like me, who naturally had optimistic tendencies, live there most of the time? *Why did my expectation of good things to come sometimes waver?*

I reflected on what I consider to be the necessary ingredients, or core components, of optimism, and then recalled times during which my own optimistic tendencies flowed like a river in spate — as well as the times when they didn't. As I mentioned earlier, optimism, like other facets of outlook, is generally stable throughout adult life — that is, as long as we don't actively try to change. However, research also shows that things such as a scarcity of resources, which I'll describe in more detail later, can temporarily change how we feel, behave, and even think during times of extreme adversity. My own experience was no different.

One work situation in particular highlights these attitudinal ups and downs. When I first came to the University of Pittsburgh as an Assistant Professor of Medicine, I had a dream to implement sweeping changes for the way cigarette smoking was treated. While smoking is the number one cause of preventable death in the U.S. and the world, and is recognized as a major risk factor for heart disease, stroke, and certain cancers, it is still erroneously considered by many health care providers as "merely a bad habit," to quote Dr. Michael Fiore, the lead architect of the current Department of Health and Human Services guidelines on treating tobacco use. What does that all mean? In many of the health care systems across the country, smoking is grossly undertreated because it doesn't fall neatly into place like other risk factors and diseases.

For example, if a patient with hypertension or diabetes walks into a clinic, the doctor addresses that patient's condition and automatically takes steps to reduce his or her risk of future heart attack and death. This may entail prescribing an aspirin, blood pressure medication, and statin medication to reduce cholesterol, and giving lifestyle advice. And insurance companies reimburse the doctor for the visit and recognize the hypertension or diabetes as a condition that requires sustained treatment for the duration of the condition, which can be decades or even lifelong.

However, this is not always the case for the roughly one in five American adults who smoke. When a patient who smokes walks into a clinic, especially if that patient is "apparently healthy," like Helen was, it is up to the individual patient or the individual doctor to address the smoking. In other words, the standard of care that applies to other chronic conditions is lagging for treating

91

smoking, and many insurance providers to date have not systematically reimbursed for the treatment of the condition in a way that helps smokers quit and stay smoke-free. Meanwhile, cigarette smoking is driving a large — if not the largest — portion of preventable death in the U.S. and the world. For many smokers, proper therapy requires multiple rounds of treatment over several years — a model I am currently studying in veterans who smoke. Fortunately, new standards and new legislation such as the Family Smoking Prevention and Tobacco Control Act are now helping the treatment of smoking catch up to that of other chronic health conditions.

But back then, things in my hospital system weren't that much different from the rest of the nation. While I had worked closely with my division chief, Dr. Wishwa Kapoor, to do more for patients who smoked, it was an arduous process to get started, and everything I tried initially failed. In my third year on faculty, we opened a clinic called Kick the Habit. The clinic closed after about a year and a half due to the combination of low attendance and preemptive economic maneuvers taken by the hospital in the wake of the 2007–2008 market crash. A big problem, which was not unique to our system, was financial. Who was going to pay for the dedicated smoking cessation counselors?

At the time, the prevailing sentiment was that while the idea of a dedicated quit-smoking service had merit, the funds simply were not there. "Besides," a colleague admonished me after one meeting, "the responsibility for quitting rests with the individual patients." (Given that cigarette smoking is an addiction, that approach is like waiting for the alcohol-dependent individual to stop drinking on his own, or the depressed person to fix herself, without any external structure or guidance.) Compelled to try and change this way of thinking, I toiled for a couple more years, largely unsuccessfully. My usual resilience was wearing thin, and I began to lose hope that a dedicated tobacco treatment service would ever materialize. Seeing no point, I actually abandoned the project for several years, but in the meantime kept in contact with one of my mentors, Dr. Nancy Rigotti, professor of medicine at Harvard Medical School and director of the Tobacco Treatment Service at Massachusetts General Hospital. I had worked with Nancy during my time in Boston as a research fellow, where she and others taught me to design clinical trials for smoking cessation. With the help of her administrators and some stellar counselors, she had built a successful quit-smoking program, which was now a model for hospitals across the nation. I remember thinking to myself on more than one occasion, "If only she were here at my institution, I would be able to get this done." Then one day it dawned on me: Why not team up with her from a distance? The very thought of having a seasoned partner in this daunting task — one who not only espoused the same goals but also had accomplished them — instantly removed a weight from my shoulders and I snapped out of my funk. The following year we submitted a multisite grant to the NIH, which ultimately was funded, and the program gained hospital-wide support as well as approval from Dr. Steven Shapiro, our chief medical and scientific officer.

Looking back, that period took quite a toll on my adrenal glands (lots of adrenaline release!). I knew that thousands of people across the region — not to mention the world — were not getting the treatment they needed for their smoking habit. Considering that more than half of smokers die prematurely from a smoking-related illness, I knew many of these people were heading to early graves. I kept wondering, though, *Why did I have to struggle so much to maintain an optimistic outlook toward achieving my goal — why not just believe in it and keep at it?* My internal struggle almost cost me my dream, because it allowed me to temporarily give up. One reason: I simply lacked the resources, including finances and at times encouragement and moral support, to pursue my vision. *New York Times* columnist David Brooks said it best when he summarized recent research on the cyclical ebb and flow of money, worry, and attention in a July 2011 piece: "Scarcity creates its own psychology." In my case, the scarcity of dollars combined with the broader medical system's initial reluctance to address smoking as a chronic condition stifled my ability to keep my eyes optimistically on the prize. But fortunately, I eventually found the tangible support of my friends and colleagues, which proved to be the antidote to my transient hopelessness by giving me enough stamina to keep working for change.

Whether you have pragmatic, incremental, struggling, or another type of optimistic tendency, or even if you don't feel you have *any* optimistic tendencies, remember that there are as many faces of optimism as there are optimists, because expecting good things to come manifests a little bit differently for each one of us. We each need to (and *can*) find one that suits us, as our optimal physical, emotional, and spiritual health may depend on it.

MY RECIPE FOR OPTIMISM PIE

We can start by identifying some of the key components that enable us to occupy more hopeful territory, at least some of the time. In the next chapter, I'll introduce some tools you can use to gauge your attitude latitude. I've thought a lot about the question of how an optimist comes to expect good things in the future. What's clear at this point is that no one knows the formula for sure. But I can describe what my own struggles have taught me about the core ingredients of *my* optimistic and pessimistic tendencies. By comparing experiences during which I was able to mobilize all the ingredients to those in which I lacked one or more of these key components, I have come up with the following list: confidence, resources (which here *very* broadly include financial, social, educational, and other types), keeping at least part of one's attention on the positive, conviction, and endurance. For me, these ingredients have produced peak optimism experiences during which I've managed to focus on my picture of future success *and* to persist in creatively pursuing that plan despite numerous barriers. Essentially, what I'm describing is my own process of problem solving, but one that plays out similarly with many people. The end result is that I've brought my future vision of success right into the now. When one or more ingredients are lacking, the optimism pie is not as sweet, but it can still come together over time, as I just described in the example of my work situation. (For a time I was not able to mobilize the resources to get the treatment service going, but I didn't permanently lose my conviction that it was important or worth pursuing.) Some of these key ingredients may emanate from each other: For example, greater confidence comes from past successes or, alternatively, from a resource safety net, whatever form that takes. Having more resources usually, but not always, resolves problems more quickly.

SCHOOL SUPPLIES: EDUCATIONAL RESOURCES

My medical (educational) training taught me that the shortness of breath, near-fainting, and other symptoms that used to frighten me as a kid (which I suffered as a result of my then-undiagnosed congenital heart condition) can usually be treated by following established algorithms. The more I put that information into practice, the more hopefully I approached even the most dire patient situations. This meant that medically, I had a good idea of what the best possible outcome would be, given the particulars of each person and each situation. It also goes without saying that educational resources do not only come from a degree — any experience we learn from adds to our educational capital.

Case in point: I remember one night on call as a resident when I was paged around one a.m. with two simultaneous codes — medical parlance for emergencies — on opposite sides of the hospital. One code is usually more than enough for anyone, including me, to handle. With two at once I shifted into overdrive and quickly triaged. I left my more experienced intern at the first patient's bedside while I sprinted off with the other intern to see the second patient, who was severely hypotensive (having dangerously low blood pressure). The nurse was having trouble with the pulse oximeter, a bedside device measuring the amount of oxygen in the blood, which also reads the heart rate. While I called for blood and prepared to place a central line, a large IV to the superior vena cava, I checked the pulse ox probe on my own finger. It was working just fine, and instantly the numbers read out: oxygen saturation 99 percent, heart rate 60 beats per minute. The nurse came over and gave me a high five. "Go, Dr. Tindle!" Even after the electrifying events of the previous few minutes, my heart was skipping along at an easy pace. At that moment, my physiology reflected my underlying experience of confidence: I knew I would get these two people safely to the next sunrise.

OUR OUTLOOK CAN CYCLE WITH OUR STRUGGLES

Just like my educational resources allowed smooth(er) sailing during that night, other types of resources, such as having money in the bank, can also serve as great buffers. While not all optimists are rich and not all pessimists are poor, there is evidence that money may grease the wheels of hopefulness, likely by reducing numerous stressors and allowing us to worry less about things that may go wrong and focus more on what we want to do. We'll discuss this further in chapter 8. Research is now demonstrating how scarcity — of money, time, and other resources — is intimately tied to another important resource we humans possess: our attention. As much as we may want to pay attention to more than one thing at a time, our brains are not designed for this. When we attempt to do two things at once, which requires us to attend to, or think about, two things at once, we actually slow down in thinking about and completing both tasks. Scarcity may exacerbate this process.

Drs. Eldar Shafir of Princeton and Sendhil Mullainathan of Harvard tested the IQs of Indian farmers before and after their harvest — times when their finances were maximally depleted and maximally flush, respectively. Before the harvest, as a consequence of being strapped for cash, the farmers were in a general state of worry, and their IQ tests were significantly lower than after the harvest, when the money flowed more freely and the farmers did not have to attend to their financial concerns moment-to-moment. The implication is that the attentional resources of these farmers — in other words, their ability to focus — were depleted by their financial worries. The fact that the IQ of each farmer cycled with the seasons illustrates the power of these mental processes, and shows us that even IQ, which we have been taught is unchanging, is in fact changeable according to our state of mind. Drs. Shafir and Mullainathan replicated these principles by studying another type of scarcity, severe lack of time, in Princeton undergraduates, demonstrating that the "consequences of having too little" can affect rich and poor people alike. While the study tested for changes in IQ (and not in optimism — the expectation of a positive future), it's easy to see why it may be harder to focus on future success during periods of scarcity, when one's attention may be pulled in myriad directions.

ATTENDING TO THE POSITIVE

In addition to confidence and resources, keeping one's eye on the positive aspects of a scenario might be necessary to expect the best outcome. Sometimes, choosing to *not* focus on the negative (or the full range of possibilities) is a blessing, because it protects us from being paralyzed by the fear that naturally arises on facing the unfiltered gravitas of a tough scenario. At the time I was undergoing heart surgery, my relative ignorance of what could go wrong medically allowed me to maintain a hopeful outlook instead of lapsing into anxiety and despair. Optimists do not propel themselves forward by ignorance, of course; we've already seen that the opposite is true.

(Veteran research psychologist Dr. Suzanne Segerstrom, author of *Breaking Murphy's Law: How Optimists Get What They Want from Life — and Pessimists Can Too* has shown that optimists tend to focus on the positive aspects of a situation, a phenomenon that she has suggested may help explain why optimists tend to adjust better. Psychologists call such a preference of focus an attentional bias — not to be confused with the optimistic bias, which we've already seen is akin to denial). In fact, there are many instances when people are fully aware of the dangers that lay ahead, but they expect good things anyway, and are determined to see those good things through because of their conviction.

My expectation to have a good outcome after surgery in turn motivated me to take steps to help myself heal — steps that I otherwise may not have taken. It didn't even occur to me that I wouldn't recover, so I behaved as if I would, and in turn did the very things that would help ensure the best outcome. I started a regular exercise program, which improved my heart's pump function and the health of my blood vessels, planned a summer vacation along La Ruta Maya throughout Central America — something to look forward to — and then got a job as a temp at a commercial real estate leasing company in Chicago's Loop to pay for the trip. Coworkers helped keep my spirits up, and even threw me a send-off party. Incidentally, I was unwittingly mobilizing and expanding my existing social network. Social support — one's connectedness with others, which is linked to better health outcomes — is another resource optimists tend to have a lot of, which we'll talk more about in chapter 5.

IKIGAI . . . ER, LIVING WITH CONVICTION

Recall *ikigai,* the Japanese concept of living life with purpose, which I introduced in chapter 1, and how those who strongly endorse *ikigai* live longer than those who do not. Conviction is what helps us avoid paralysis and face our fear when the shield of ignorance is gone. Dr. Martin Luther King Jr., who had already survived a stabbing and been threatened repeatedly when he delivered his "But, if not" sermon at the Ebenezer Baptist Church in Atlanta in November 1967, is an example of such intense conviction, and I've often looked to his words to help me focus on the *quality* of my life, and not just the length of it:

You may be 38 years old, as I happen to be. And one day, some great opportunity stands before you and calls you to stand up for some great principle, some great issue, some great cause. And you refuse to do it because you are afraid. . . . You refuse to do it because you want to live longer. . . . Well you may go on and live until you are 90, but you're just as dead at 38 as you would be at 90. And the cessation of breathing in your life is but the belated announcement of an earlier death of the spirit.

Dr. King illustrates as no one else can how physical health isn't the only goal: There is also the critical health of the spirit, which applies to all of us whether we are religiously affiliated or not. When we pursue our calling, and what makes us truly happy, even if we can only spend part of our time doing so, we live better, healthier lives. By contrast, when we turn away from what gives us joy, the road we travel is one of drudgery and emptiness. Soon after that speech, in his prophetic "I've been to the mountaintop" address in Memphis, Tenn., Dr. King underscored the importance of moving forward in the face of uncertainty.

Well, I don't know what will happen now. We've got some difficult days ahead. But it really doesn't matter with me now, because I've been to the mountaintop. And I don't mind. Like anybody, I would like to live a long life. Longevity has its place. But I'm not concerned about that now. I just want to do God's will.

For Dr. King, the goal of equality was personal as well as universal. For the rest of us, a goal may be less grand, but it is meaningful nonetheless, especially when we approach it with conviction.

People find meaning in many places — nature, religion, travel, love — and our goals don't necessarily have to be lofty. They just have to be real enough to us that we want to pursue them. An optimistic outlook is key in that it points us in the direction we naturally want to go — not necessarily because we are trying to get good at something but because *we want to do it.* When we envision good things around the bend, we are motivated to persist in working toward them, and are thus more likely to obtain them. This isn't just wishful thinking; it's science. Evidence from one neuroimaging study, led by Dr. Tali Sharot, author of *The*

Optimism Bias: A Tour of the Irrationally Positive Brain, showed that when optimists imagine positive events in the future, such as a reunion with a loved one, they demonstrate greater brain activity than pessimists in key areas of the limbic system, a major brain network responsible for thinking and feeling. Translation: Optimists may be able to envision a bright future more vividly, and embrace it with greater tenacity. Nobody gets to the proverbial mountaintop by believing that they can't (and therefore don't) start walking. In this sense, as we saw with Helen at the beginning of her journey, being afraid to hope could cost you your health and many years of your life.

Strengthening our own sense of purpose may also affect us at the cellular level, as we saw with the study on meditation and telomeres in the previous chapter. If cultivating your own sense of purpose is key to healthy aging, how do you go about doing it?

In the following chapters, I'll show you a number of ways my friends, colleagues, patients, and I have managed to find varying degrees of success in this arena.

ENDURING OPTIMISTS

Staying optimistic may ultimately require marathon endurance through desolate times. During my own difficult times I have relied on the inspiring example set by Mother Teresa, arguably one of the most dedicated individuals of the twentieth century, who continued her mission to alleviate the suffering of the poor, ill, and disenfranchised in India despite her own serious doubts that she had any connection to the divine. In one of her letters in 1953, which was made public posthumously despite her wish for privacy, she revealed the feeling of being cut off from God:

> Please pray specially for me that I may not spoil His work and that Our Lord may show Himself — for there is such terrible darkness within me, as if everything was dead. It has been like this more or less from the time I started "the work."

So the message for the rest of us struggling optimists is: If the great ones sometimes falter, then the rest of us shouldn't feel bad when we do. We all struggle to varying extents. The important thing is to not give up. Mother Teresa's doubts — the knowledge of which I consider to be a gift to humanity — demonstrate that she did not wake up and float out of her humble bed every morning propelled effortlessly by the certainty of union with God. On the contrary, she wrestled with her daily doubts, yet showed up to work anyway, and very concretely delivered her own vision of grace to the world.

For those of us who acknowledge the benefits of an optimistic outlook but still struggle to maintain one, the take-home point is this: Even the brightest bulbs sometimes flicker. Being an optimist doesn't necessarily mean you're the brightest bulb on the Christmas tree. It means you keep your bulb burning brightly and steadily enough to light up your own path — and maybe the path of others — to better physical, mental, and spiritual health.

3
THE SAVVY OUTLOOK
TRAVELER 1: PREPARATION

How do you know if your outlook could use a nudge in any particular direction? Put simply, if your current perspective is preventing you from heartily following the steps to healthy aging that I've already outlined, change could do you good. That means that most of us, myself included, can benefit from some outlook orienteering. Sometimes our "outlook barriers" are not immediately obvious and can live with us unseen for years until circumstances unearth them. We saw a perfect example of this in the previous chapter with my patient Helen, who was well into her sixties before realizing that she was "worth taking care of," as she put it. Prior to that, she had lived life with the tacit understanding that she was not worth the effort. This belief, conspiring with her fatalistic view of a future that offered no change from the present — meaning that she would forever be subject to the erratic whims of an alcohol-dependent and abusive husband — had insidiously steered her down a dangerous road toward disability and early death. Only after becoming aware of how her outlook was keeping her down was she able to start moving up.

Even if we consider our current attitude latitude to be ideal, recall that these coordinates may vary with circumstances. Myriad scarcities, including lack of social support, tight finances, and sleep deprivation, affect our psychology and may temporarily blow us off course. When caught in such squalls, how do we identify the resources we need and reorient ourselves in order to either maintain or regain a healthy position? And what if we find ourselves in scarcity mode most or all of the time? The methods I describe in this and the following chapters are meant to help you optimize your outlook, whether you are looking to do so for a particular challenge or to make more sweeping change. Baby steps are OK, and you should move at a pace that is comfortable for you.

To provide a path, I've organized data from medical research and the crucible of my own experiences as a physician and a patient into the 7 **Steps of Attitudinal Change.**

1. Determine your current attitude latitude (Point A)
2. Aim your brain in the desired direction (Point B): Form an intention to change
3. Examine your outlook in action by learning to listen to your inner conversation
4. Acknowledge your accomplishments along the way
5. Follow typical doctor advice
6. Reach out for the benefits of social support
7. Get a healthy dose of green: Cultivate your microenvironment

This chapter focuses on steps 1 and 2. Chapter 4 is dedicated to step 3, and chapter 5 explains steps 4 through 7, which provide new impetus to follow "typical doctor advice." In one sense, outlook travel is no different than regular travel. To get from **Point A** (your current attitude latitude) to **Point B** (the attitude latitude you'd like to occupy), it helps if you know a little about the terrain of each territory and get a feel for how they differ before you set out. You'll also need to plan for a means of transportation and the energy to power your trip.

Step 1: Determine your current attitude lati-

tude using a few questionnaires commonly employed by psychologists. This process will illustrate aspects of where your Point A is, helping you appreciate your unique outlook.

Step 2: Learn to "aim your brain" in the desired direction (Point B) by forming an intention to enhance or diminish certain aspects of your outlook. To aim your brain, you must have at least some degree of openness and curiosity about the big wide outlook world, and you may want to adopt an attitude that is even more open, more optimistic, less angry, or otherwise different from your current perspective.

Your intention is like the gas in your car, the wind in your sails, or the glycogen in your liver: It fuels your journey.

Before we begin, I want to make two points. First, there is no single path to a healthier outlook. These seven steps are meant to serve as guideposts to help you reach your desired outlook destination. In the process of following them, you may find some of your own landmarks. Second, sometimes we don't change our attitude latitude deliberately, or in stepwise fashion, so you may find yourself beginning with one of the later steps, which is perfectly fine. In the first chapter I spoke of a frame shift, in which circumstances such as a major life event (lung cancer) may blow us with gale-force winds into a whole new perspective (quitting smoking goes from impossible to possible). Other times, in the absence of obvious precipitating circumstances, we simply start doing something differently — maybe buying a new pair of running shoes and exercising every day after work with a friend — and this new action is the first in a string of changes that over time allow us to see things from a new vantage point. I'll talk more about this in chapter 5 when we discuss exercise, sleep, and other behaviors. My teacher and friend Franciscan priest and activist Father Richard Rohr recognizes this way of attitudinal change: "We don't think ourselves into new ways of living. We live ourselves into new ways of thinking." For those of us who have not been shocked into change by life-altering circumstances or are not currently living ourselves into a new outlook, following these steps is a smart place to start.

STEP 1: DETERMINE YOUR ATTITUDE LATITUDE (POINT A)

The three questionnaires that will help you identify your Point A are by no means an exhaustive battery, but represent some of the main scales that I've used in my own research and that factor into other research that I describe. The first is the Life Orientation Test, Revised (LOT-R), designed to provide a general idea of your overall degree of optimism or pessimism and, as you now know, predict many aspects of health and aging, including risk of heart attack, stroke, and death. Keep in mind it does not illuminate the nuances that may be unique to you, whether you are "pragmatic," "incremental," or "struggling," or have some other personal twist on the general character trait of optimism. Recall that I created these subcategories, which are not part of the research literature, to help you "see your own face" in this amazing character trait.

The second questionnaire taps into self-compassion — a way of relating to ourselves that is built on kindness, understanding, and emotional balance. Self-compassion, which we'll talk more about in chapter 6, has been linked to better self-care and healthier behaviors. This unique scale was developed by Dr. Kristin Neff, associate professor in human development and culture at the University of Texas at Austin and author of *Self-Compassion: Stop Beating Yourself Up and Leave Insecurity Behind*. Dr. Neff explains that self-compassion "entails being warm and understanding toward ourselves when we suffer, fail, or feel inadequate, rather than ignoring our pain or flagellating ourselves with self-criticism." She describes how having compassion for oneself is just like having compassion for other people. In order to be truly compassionate, we must first notice suffering, empathize with the sufferer, and recognize that suffering is universal. Each of these three facets of compassion keeps the experience from spilling over into pity or overidentification with any specific situation or circumstance. In the chapters that follow I'll introduce some techniques, including mindfulness and contemplation, that naturally support compassion.

The third questionnaire assesses the Big Five traits introduced in chapter 1: neuroticism, extroversion, openness, conscientiousness, and agreeableness. As I noted, each of these traits has been linked to our sense of well-being, health behaviors, and healthy aging.

For all three questionnaires, there are no right or wrong answers and no single score threshold that automatically sets you in lush paradise or banishes you to barren wasteland on planet Outlook. The intention of this exercise is to provide one way of seeing yourself. When I first filled out the LOT-R (the first questionnaire, which I've included next for you), I did not score as very optimistic, which may reflect my tendency to struggle to be hopeful. For these orientation tools to be effective, you must put your true foot forward and resist the urge to contort yourself to fit into another person's shoes (including the person you may want to be). So as you answer the questions, put aside any notions about Cinderella's perfect glass slipper.

1. Optimism

Please be as honest and accurate as you can throughout. Try not to let your response to one statement influence your responses to other statements. There are no correct or incorrect answers. Answer according to your own feelings, rather than how you think most people would answer.

1 Strongly Disagree
2 Disagree
3 Neutral
4 Agree
5 Strongly Agree

_____1. In uncertain times, I usually expect the best.

_____2. If something can go wrong for

116

me, it will.

_____3. I'm always optimistic about my future.

_____4. I hardly ever expect things to go my way.

_____5. I rarely count on good things happening to me.

_____6. Overall, I expect more good things to happen to me than bad.

Scoring and Interpretation: To score, first subtotal the answers to questions 1, 3, and 6. Questions 2, 4, and 5 are reverse-scored, meaning that a 1 is scored as a 5 and a 2 is scored as a 4 (3 remains a 3). Once you've reverse-scored these three questions, subtotal them and add this to the first subtotal for your final score. The higher you score on the LOT-R, the more optimistic your outlook. Unlike scales for depression or other clinical conditions, there is no cut point or threshold for being optimistic or pessimistic. However, in my own work with older adults, those who scored below 22 tended to be more pessimistic, while those who scored 26 or higher tended to be more optimistic. In clinical populations, such as people who have medical conditions, all scores tend to be lower than in healthier populations, as you might expect.

M. F. Scheier, C. S. Carver, and M. W. Bridges, "Distinguishing Optimism from Neuroticism (and Trait Anxiety, Self-Master, and Self-Esteem): A Reevaluation of the Life Orientation Test," *Journal of Personality and Social Psychology* 67, no. 6 (1994): 1063–78.

2. Self-Compassion (How I Typically Act Toward Myself in Difficult Times)

Please read each statement carefully before answering. To the left of each item, indicate how often you behave in the stated manner.

For the first set of items, use the following scale:

Almost never 1 2 3 4 5 Almost always

_____I try to be understanding and patient toward those aspects of my personality I don't like.

_____When something painful happens I try to take a balanced view of the situation.

_____I try to see my failings as part of the human condition.

_____When I'm going through a very hard time, I give myself the caring and tenderness I need.

118

_____When something upsets me I try to keep my emotions in balance.

_____When I feel inadequate in some way, I try to remind myself that feelings of inadequacy are shared by most people.

For the next items, use the following scale (notice the endpoints of the scale differ from above):

Almost always 1 2 3 4 5 Almost never

_____When I fail at something important to me I become consumed by feelings of inadequacy.

_____When I'm feeling down, I tend to feel like most other people are probably happier than I am.

_____When I fail at something that's important to me, I tend to feel alone in my failure.

_____When I'm feeling down I tend to obsess and fixate on everything that's wrong.

_____I'm disapproving and judgmental about my own flaws and inadequacies.

_____I'm intolerant and impatient toward those aspects of my personality I don't like.

Total (sum of all 12 items)_____
Average score (Total divided by 12)_____

Average overall self-compassion scores tend to be around 3.0 on the 1–5 scale, so you can interpret your overall score accordingly. As a rough guide, a score of 1–2.5 indicates you are low in self-compassion, 2.5–3.5 is moderate, and 3.5–5.0 is high.

F. Raes, E. Pommier, K. D. Neff, and D. Van Gucht, "Construction and Factorial Validation of a Short Form of the Self-Compassion Scale," *Clinical Psychology and Psychotherapy* 18, no. 3 (2011): 250–55.

3. The "Big Five" Personality Traits
The next questions are phrases describing people's behaviors. Please use the rating scale below to describe how accurately each statement describes you, and then mark the box that corresponds with your answer. Describe yourself as you generally are now, not as you wish to be in the future.

1 Very Inaccurate
2 Moderately Inaccurate
3 Neutral
4 Moderately Accurate
5 Very Accurate

_____1. Am the life of the party.

_____2. Sympathize with others' feelings.

_____3. Get chores done right away.

_____4. Have frequent mood swings.

_____5. Have a vivid imagination.

_____6. Don't talk a lot.

_____7. Am not interested in other people's problems.

_____8. Often forget to put things back in their proper place.

_____9. Am relaxed most of the time.

_____10. Am not interested in abstract ideas.

_____11. Talk to a lot of different people at parties.

_____12. Feel others' emotions.

_____13. Like order.

_____14. Get upset easily.

_____15. Have difficulty understanding abstract ideas.

_____16. Keep in the background.

_____17. Am not really interested in others.

_____18. Make a mess of things.

_____19. Seldom feel blue.

_____20. Do not have a good imagination.

Scoring and Interpretation: Bear with me here — the scoring may seem tricky, but it's not as complicated as it looks. For each of the following 5 scales, you will need to reverse-score some of the questions, so a 1 is scored as a 5 and a 2 is scored as a 4 (3 remains a 3). Then sum all four questions for that scale and divide by 4. You're done! Each of these five scales yields a score from 1 to 5, where 1 is low on that trait and 5 is high. So for example, if I'm a 5 on extroversion, I am an extrovert. If I am a 3 on openness, I have moderate openness to new experiences (neither high nor low). Note that you do *not* add up all the items together for a grand total. (Instead, you have a total for each of the 5 scales.)

Extroversion scale: Questions 1, 6, 11, 16. Reverse the scores on questions 6 and 16.

Agreeableness scale: Questions 2, 7, 12, 17. Reverse the scores on questions 7 and 17.

Conscientiousness scale: Questions 3, 8, 13, 18. Reverse the scores on questions 8 and 18.

Neuroticism scale: Questions 4, 9, 14, 19. Reverse the scores on questions 9 and 19.

Openness/imaginativeness scale: Questions 5, 10, 15, 20. Reverse the scores on questions 10 and 15.

M. B. Donnellan, F. L. Oswald, B. M. Baird, R. E. Lucas, "The Mini-IPIP Scales: Tiny-yet-effective measures of the Big Five Factors of Personality." *Psychological Assessment* 18(2), June 2006: 192–203.

Now that you've mapped some of your traits, what do you think of your Point A? Did you land on the "X" as predicted, or were there any surprises? What was your internal reaction upon learning your coordinates? I cannot stress enough how our outlook coordinates are the product of multiple traits. We are not black-and-white stick figures but, rather, multidimensional creatures sporting a spectrum of shades in between; we all have degrees of optimism, pessimism, self-compassion, conscientiousness, and many other facets. Nor are we necessarily stuck in the attitude latitude of our birth and our youth, although we certainly could stay there, and most people do.

Equally important to consider is that you may not have to travel very far on the outlook globe to reach a desired destination

— to become more optimistic, less self-critical, or less angry, for example. In chapters 6 and 7 I'll discuss how even small differences in attitude latitude can have big consequences for health and aging, meaning that people who differ by only one point on the attitude scales have measurable differences in their risk of disease and death. I'll also show you how one man's outlook journey — which involved a few key shifts in openness and optimism — changed the course of his own life and the lives of his children and grandchildren, and influenced hundreds of his students and colleagues, including me.

STEP 2: AIM YOUR BRAIN TOWARD POINT B: FORM AN INTENTION TO CHANGE

Having established Point A, you now want to give yourself a clear direction toward Point B. Where would you like to go? Which aspects of your outlook would you like to enhance or diminish? And what will inspire you to get there? Changing our outlook in the service of healthy aging is a compelling motivator. As one coworker in her fifties told me after learning about a study on exercise and memory (which I'll describe in chapter 5), "If walking every day keeps my brain's hippocampus from shrinking and my memory sharp, you can be damned sure I'm open to walking every day." Yet motivation is highly idiosyncratic, and the answer to "Why should I bother?" is not the same for everyone.

In fact, much of the time, our primary intention may not be to change our outlook, but rather to change something else that is important to us — something that just so happens to be linked to outlook. For example, did you even care much about your outlook before you learned how it could affect your aging? When we realize how our current outlook coordinates hinder us from accomplishing something we care about, we allow ourselves the option of seeing things differently, and we become outlook travelers. Take a moment to consider your own intention(s): *What do you want to change, and why?*

The intention, or purpose, behind any path you take is just as important as the steps you take on that path. To understand the incredible power of intention from a biological perspective, consider the latest research on motor neuroprosthetics — robotic arms that paralyzed people are using to drink coffee, type on a keyboard, and to literally reach out to loved ones, among

other activities of daily living. Neuroprosthetics are initiated by the quadriplegic or
paraplegic's own brain waves. We don't usually think about what goes on in our brain
when we put our mind to something, like
reaching out to turn on the light. Yet every
action begins with an intention, which in
our brain is the first in a series of actual
biochemical events that eventually generate
enough energy to move an arm, be it flesh
or metal. It's worth noting that when a
person first begins using a neuroprosthetic,
it can take days or weeks for him to learn to
use it effectively. First he must focus his attention on a task, and then practice, over
and over, turning that intention into action.

As outlook travelers, we are not trying to
move prosthetic limbs, although changing
our outlook may literally get us moving in
healthier directions. Instead of aiming our
electrical brain impulses into our motor
cortex — the area of the brain initiating the
signal to move our limbs — we are aiming
our electrical impulses into the brain regions
that govern how we think and feel. In this
sense, we can "decide" to think and feel a
certain way. This does not mean that we are
seeking control over every thought or feeling. Instead, we are learning to *aim* our
thoughts and feelings toward a given target.

When we intend to do something, we are directing the neurochemical impulses from our frontal cortex, a key decision-making area, to guide neurochemical impulses in other regions of our brain, such as the limbic system, that underlie thinking and feeling.

Before you decide that aiming your brain is too complicated, know that you have already done it a million times! You did it when you learned to crawl, walk, and run. Every time you learn something, no matter how small, your brain aims and actually changes. It's called *neuroplasticity,* which refers to the process by which neurons change and make new connections with each other. You may have heard or read of neuroplasticity before, but have you considered just how adept you are at this remarkable process? Practice repeatedly, and you strengthen the intention, just as the paraplegics practiced aiming their brains into their prostheses to be able to move again. Whether we are formulating and executing our intention to crawl, move a neuroprosthetic, or undertake outlook travel, the process requires focus, practice, encouragement, and reward.

If intention isn't something you've thought much about, it's important to understand that without it, our actions may lose steam and peter out altogether, or never get started in the first place. Here's an example of how a clear intention is key to aligning outlook and action toward healthy aging. I recently met Joseph, a man who joined one of my research studies to quit smoking. He had started smoking when he joined the military shortly after high school, and now in his early sixties, he was really feeling his age. He had developed chronic obstructive pulmonary disease (COPD), was now having progressive breathing difficulty, and even had to carry around a portable oxygen tank.

His declining health worried him, but it became clear that at its core, it was not because he feared death or disability for its own sake, but because he might leave his elderly mother without a caregiver. Yet the stress of caring for her day in and day out was overwhelming him, as it does many people in his position, and he repeatedly succumbed to the urge to smoke despite a strong desire to quit. As we worked with Joseph over several months, it was clear that he was burning out, a fact that he acknowledged but that he would not take steps to ameliorate. Interestingly, his lack of action was not due to lack of resources: He had another family member who was able and willing to provide respite care, and he had the financial coverage to bring his mother to adult community activities for a couple of hours each week. (Respite care, even for a short time, is critical for the well-being of a primary caregiver.) Joseph was on a dangerous track that he either couldn't or wouldn't get off of, and we had to help him find another path.

Like many smokers, Joseph was also reluctant to use nicotine replacement — the patch, gum, lozenges, etc. — to help him resist the smoking urges. Then during one visit, while he reiterated his concern for his mother's welfare if he were not there, the counselor pointed out something obvious yet powerful: The best way for Joseph to care for his mother was to keep *himself* healthy, and by far the most effective way to do that was to quit smoking. Even in older adults who have smoked for decades, quitting smoking substantially improves breathing, halves the risk of heart attack within a year, and lowers the risk of dying. Just as we saw earlier with Helen, it really is never too late. The most effective way to quit smoking, in turn, was to keep seeing the counselor, temporarily use the nicotine-replacement medication to help him weather cravings, and get some backup at home to reduce his overall stress level. We all saw the lightbulb go on in Joseph's mind as he nodded in agreement with the plan. The counselor's observation had helped Joseph align his intention — to do whatever it took to protect his mother — with his action: quitting smoking. Simply realizing how these pieces fit together catapulted him into new outlook territory, because in this most important of life situations, his perspective had changed. That same day, Joseph got a relief caregiver and began using the nicotine patch.

Intention is especially critical when we are divided. Sometimes our inner traits are at odds with each other, and we must choose to foster one over the other. In *Taking the Leap: Freeing Ourselves from Old Habits and Fears,* Buddhist monk Pema Chödrön relates a widely known Native American legend of the two wolves, this time applied to a modern-day scenario. A grandfather describes to his grandson his nuanced reaction to the September 11, 2001, attacks: a mixture of bloodthirsty rage and deep compassion for the victims. He likens this internal struggle to two wolves fighting in his heart — one wolf is angry and vengeful, the other gentle and compassionate. The two are equally matched in strength, agility, and cunning. The young boy asks his grandfather which wolf will win the battle. His response: "Whichever one I feed." Coming back to attitudes, each wolf represents an aspect of our outlook that may be vying for our attention. So how do we feed one inner wolf over the other? *We formulate the intention to do so.*

Clinical psychologist David Bresler and physician Marty Rossman, my guided imagery teachers, always said that whatever you put your attention on grows. It may surprise you to consider that simply focusing your attention on different aspects of the same situation can plant seeds to shift your outlook. To illustrate this concept with the traits of optimism and pessimism, I asked optimism world expert and lead author of the LOT-R, Dr. Michael Scheier, to help us out with a scenario he relates to his students.

Damn, I've Won the Lottery!

"It's like this," Dr. Scheier says, smiling jovially. "An optimist and a pessimist both win the lottery. The optimist says, 'Hey, this is fantastic, I won all this money!' The pessimist snarls, 'Damn it, now I have to pay all these taxes!' " Objectively speaking, both of them are correct. It's just a matter of where they choose to focus their attention. Dr. Scheier further illustrates this with a twist on the familiar glass half-empty or half-full metaphor. "If you ask people to point to the water level, everyone points to the same line in the glass — both optimists and pessimists know where it is. The question is, what does it *mean* to them?" So neither optimists nor pessimists are factually right or wrong, but their focus and interpretation do have consequences for their moment-to-moment experience, which, as we've seen, directly and indirectly influences health and aging. I've already described how I tend to straddle the fence between an optimistic and a pessimistic outlook, depending on my circumstances, and were it not for my conscious intention to "feed the optimistic wolf," I could just as easily fall off on either side. In practice this means actively monitoring my perspective and making an intention to grab hold of the more hopeful thoughts that well up, while noticing and letting go of the more fatalistic ones.

It's an ongoing surveillance process, and it takes work. Over time, as fatalistic thoughts emerge, I've learned to recognize them, at least some of the time, as part of an old script that I no longer wish to follow.

These thoughts also tend to cycle in predictable patterns, sort of like a rainy season over my outlook territory, when I am particularly short on sleep, time, or both, such as before a major project deadline. During these tough times my brain conjures not only the anxiety surrounding the deadline itself, but a whole slew of other, unrelated problems — other unfinished projects, past scenarios of every kind in which I didn't do my best work, the fact that I haven't cleaned out the garage in two years, etc. You may have experienced this ballooning of stressors, too; I refer to it as a "negativity cycle," but you may have your own label.

I've identified several methods to break this cycle, but before implementing any of these strategies, I remember my overarching intention: "At every turn, I want to think, feel, and live more optimistically." To remind myself, I wrote this down on stickies and tacked them to my computer, whiteboard, car dashboard, and other places. Once I'm hooked into my intention, my actions have more traction and are easier to implement: 1) sleep, if only for an hour; 2) exercise, if only for ten to fifteen minutes; 3) brief positive mood induction by watching YouTube clips of *Zoolander, Pulp Fiction,* and Monty Python skits; and 4) setting small goals, as in writing one paragraph for a paper or grant, or looking up one clinical fact to help a patient. Something else I find instantly reorienting is reading and listening to news reports every day, because as I hear about the details of other people's lives across the country and around the world, I am all the more thankful for my family, food, water, shelter, education and a job that allows me to apply it, and other basics that too many people lack. After hitting these reset buttons, I am often more able to see my life for the gift that it is.

We all want to feel better more often. If you find you are still unsure of precisely which direction to take your outlook, try this: Make the intention to adopt whatever attitude enhances your ability to do more of something you like to do, and your attitudinal directions will naturally follow. Starting small is a good thing. For example, I happen to love shopping at secondhand clothing stores. There's something about the thrill of finding beautiful clothing for really cheap that makes me feel good, and it also scores approval points with my ninety-two-year-old Great Depression–tested great-aunt Dorothy. It's been several years since I've visited a resale shop, even though my route home from work takes me right past a particularly enticing Goodwill store in Penn Circle. For years I've blamed this inertia on my perpetual state of time-hunger. Then one day, on my forty-second birthday, my research team went out for our annual lunch at a burger place next door to the Goodwill store, and I made the decision with two coworkers to go in (the power of social support!) . . . and I got a gorgeous summer dress with matching shoes for ten bucks. What's more, I began to think about other things I like to do — traveling, making Rick Bayless's Oaxacan black mole (an all-day affair), admiring cool bugs on the ground — and to strategize how I might do more of them. It also reminded me of some of the things I've never done but have been wanting to learn for years: double Dutch and scaling a climbing wall. I resolved to make these a reality in the next year.

This scenario may at first blush seem silly to you — having to actually make an intention to spend twenty minutes doing something that is purely joyful to you — but think about your own life and the hours in any given day. After the time claimed by your job; the needs of children, other family, friends, and pets; the time it takes to shower, brush teeth, grocery shop, etc., how much is left over? I'm guessing you said "none" or "too little." If there is any time left, how much of it are you spending on the things that make you *you*? In my case, I needed to break out of the rigid schedule rut I had lived myself into — believing that there was no time for me to take even a short detour from the day-in, day-out routine. And this is ironic, because I am pretty open and imaginative, but I had clearly become less so given my increasingly demanding schedule. Like the Indian farmers whose IQs dropped preharvest because of extreme worry about finances, I found that my typical openness to experience had narrowed due to worry about deadlines of every kind. And my self-compassion, which was just so-so to begin with, plummeted as I shoved my own needs aside in favor of the relentless completion of tasks. In the words of the poet e. e. cummings, I had "closed myself as fingers," and had to seize the opportunity, with the help of friends, to "reopen" to doing what I love. In addition to making us feel good, evidence shows that experiencing even small doses of connection and joy is beneficial for physical health. This is just one small but significant way in which the power of intention can shape our outlook, health, and aging.

In the future, we may be able to use ever

more sophisticated biofeedback methods, such as real-time fMRI (rt-fMRI), a relatively new technology that can show you a "movie" of your own brain activity. The activity of clusters of neurons in select regions of your brain is represented by a visual image: for example, a bonfire on the beach. This familiar image, and specifically the height of the flame, is a physical representation of one's brain activity in real time: Just as a true flame rises, falls, and flickers, our brain activity varies from moment to moment. Already, everyday people like you and me have participated in research studies in which they learned to use rt-fMRI to manipulate the activity of their brains with this visual biofeedback method. Several studies have focused on an area called the anterior cingulate cortex (ACC), which is key for cravings and the experience of pain. In one study, ACC activity corresponded to the degree of pain people reported feeling in response to a heat probe applied to the skin, a common experimental method to induce pain. When people "dialed up" their own ACC activity by doing mental maneuvers to increase the height of the flame on the screen, their perception of pain went up. As they dialed it down (diminishing the height of the flame), their perception of pain went down. Here's the amazing part: *The temperature of the heat probe itself never changed.* The only thing that changed was the research participants' brain activity *in response to* the heat probe. Such findings give new meaning to my suggestion to aim your brain.

You may be curious as to how people go about dialing up and dialing down their own brain activity in the scanner and in life. What are they thinking or feeling when they aim their brains in a given direction? We dial ourselves up and down all the time: Someone cuts you off in traffic and your limbic system (emotional brain) is instantly revved up. Or, you calm yourself after a heated argument by taking some deep breaths or making plans with friends. But we typically do these things unconsciously, and it may seem harder when we actually try to perform on cue. In the rt-fMRI research studies, participants were given suggestions for some common cognitive strategies, which I'll describe in detail in the next chapter. Which strategies people actually choose to deploy, and how effective each strategy may be, is beyond what the research can tell us right now. While an rt-fMRI scanner would be nice (provided you don't mind loud noises and are not claustrophobic), you do not need one to begin practicing the techniques to start looking *up*. In fact, everything you need is in your head already. Now that you've determined your Point A/current attitude latitude (step 1) and aimed your brain with an intention toward Point B/new attitude latitude (step 2), you're ready for step 3. Step 3 is examining your outlook in action, and learning to listen to the inner conversation we are having all the time with ourselves, which we may not always be aware of, and which may be leading us in ways we don't necessarily want to go.

4
THE SAVVY OUTLOOK TRAVELER 2: MOVING UP

Now we're ready to continue moving down the path with *Step 3: Examine your own outlook in action.* Here we'll learn to pay close attention to the moment-to-moment flow of thoughts and feelings comprising our inner conversation. I'll introduce you to five powerful techniques to help you drop in on this inner conversation. Learning to listen to ourselves in this way is so critical to moving *up* that I believe the skill should be instilled in us as children, right up there with math, reading, and science.

Why am I such a champion of self-examination? Consider this: Your inner conversation is an endless stream of thoughts and beliefs about *everything* — including your health, aging, and circumstances — and you may be telling yourself the darnedest things without even realizing it. We've already seen examples of how our thoughts can be barriers to healthy aging.

When we go along with thoughts such as "I will always be a failure" or "I've been overweight for so long, change doesn't matter," we sentence ourselves to unhealthy circumstances. Would you talk this way to a dear friend? Probably not. In this chapter, I invite you to observe yourself and get familiar with the unique way in which you are experiencing your own Point A. This is very important, because while you may have certain pessimistic tendencies just like the next person, they manifest according to your own life and circumstances. In other words, Point A for two different optimists or pessimists does not look exactly the same. That's why you need to go a step beyond filling out the questionnaires, pay attention to yourself, and identify the specific ways you want to change, even if you don't yet know how. Historically, all of the great teachers — religious and nonreligious, from east to west — have emphasized the importance of the "examined" life. To truly inculcate this wisdom, we must examine and understand our outlook.

I should note that for some people, step 3 — (*examining your outlook in action by learning to listen to your inner conversation*) may actually precede step 2 (*aiming your brain toward Point B through intention*), especially if you don't come to this process knowing what it is you want to change or believing that change is warranted. It may only be after taking the time to examine your outlook in close detail that you realize tweaking certain aspects may in fact help you. As far as the tools for dropping in on your own inner chitchat and redirecting it, for now it's enough to simply learn about the concepts for their own sake, before attempting to use them to get anywhere or accomplish a particular goal. This will help you take pressure off yourself to "do it right." To use a metaphor from ballroom dancing, first get a few basic steps down, then let loose and cut a rug. Or in this case, a magic outlook carpet.

STEP 3: EXAMINE YOUR OUTLOOK IN ACTION BY LEARNING TO LISTEN TO YOUR INNER CONVERSATION

We can learn to observe where we are putting our attention and eventually shift it at will in new directions. When we practice this process under the guidance of a strong intention, we begin to cultivate a new attitude. To that end, we need to come face-to-face with our own internal dialogue so that we can learn whether we truly believe the things we're telling ourselves. When you approach your thoughts and beliefs as if they were hypotheses to be proven or refuted, you become the researcher of your own case study. There are many effective methods for doing what the experts call "dropping in," but I've chosen to describe the five with which I've had direct experience, and which are supported by promising evidence: 1) cognitive behavioral therapy (CBT), 2) mindfulness, 3) contemplation, 4) guided imagery, and 5) motivational interviewing. More research has been conducted on some of these methods than others. For example, contemplation is one of the oldest practices, yet few medical studies on contemplation exist.

Each technique originates from a different tradition: CBT from Western psychotherapy, mindfulness from Buddhism, contemplation from Christianity, etc. Thanks to my mother, who exposed me to so many of the world's religions and cultural traditions, I learned some of these practices as a child. Later on, I studied them further while I was a research fellow at Harvard and on faculty at the University of Pittsburgh; working with colleagues, I have adapted two of them (guided imagery and mindfulness) for smoking cessation programs. These are techniques I have taught in my own practice, evaluated in my research studies, and just as important, incorporated into my personal routine to examine my own minute-to-minute experiences. Even if you are familiar with some or all of these techniques, practicing them in the service of changing your outlook may be new to you.

The basic idea behind any method of self-examination is that most of us actually have really good insights about our deep-seated longings, fears, desires, and beliefs. I liken these beliefs to undercurrents or seismic activity beneath our attitudinal coordinates, because they so strongly influence the terrain. Some of these undercurrents, such as "I will always be alone" or "I'm really not good enough to pull off x, y, or z task," can wait, like silent companions, for years — until we discover them by dropping in on our inner conversation and taking a closer look. We may not realize the strength of the current until it begins to sweep us away, threatening our vitality. Humans across the globe and over the eons have experienced various currents. We can learn the most by listening to those who have been pulled under, yet have managed to find their way to the surface. In September 2012, BBC correspondent Rebecca Kesby interviewed reformed members of New Zealand's most notorious and violent gangs. Growing up in abject poverty and subject to violence as children, these men firmly believed that they did not have a future. It's no surprise that many were imprisoned for violent crimes as minors, and turned to substance abuse and continued violence as part of their daily routine as young adults.

Yet many have found a way out by making new connections, both spiritually and socially, which has given them the wherewithal to evaluate their outlook and start making necessary changes. These young men display profound insight into how their fears of never attaining outward success and being societal outcasts drove their initial membership into gangs and helped feed their destructive behavior. One young man called "Jordan" has not only been able to recognize his own dangerous undercurrents but has also taken major steps to change them, mostly by having the courage to look his former attitude squarely in the eye. When asked by Kesby, "What do you think you were frightened of?" Jordan responds:

The big picture — of what you see out there in life, and how people's lives can be so glamorous. When you see people in Mercedes and BMWs, you're like, 'Is that how life is meant to be?' It was *unreachable* for us — [I was afraid] to be a failure to society. That's what [my] fear was. But now I'm on this side of the fence, with God. That's set me free. And fear has got nothing to do with it. You're someone. You've become someone.

As Helen and Jordan demonstrate, our fears and beliefs can sabotage any one of us, wherever we happen to be on the socioeconomic ladder, leading us down a path to premature disease and death. It is imperative that we master our attitudinal geography and shape it in our favor and/or move to healthier ground. Toward that end, my hope is that at least one of the following methods resonates with you.

Cognitive Behavioral Therapy (CBT)

CBT is a tool you may have heard of or used before — it's a standard method of self-examination, developed by American psychiatrist Dr. Aaron Beck, that has been proven to help people with depression, anxiety, addictions, and many other problems. CBT is usually learned and practiced with a counselor, but you don't have to have a diagnosis or an in-the-flesh therapist to benefit from it. Having utilized core CBT components with my patients, I routinely use it on myself to put my own rogue thoughts in check. In CBT, you are simply turning the spotlight on your own thoughts, feelings (and sometimes even physical sensations), identifying where these may be inaccurate or exaggerated, and then devising and implementing a plan to correct those distortions.

The most basic exercise in CBT is the "ABC" system of monitoring our thoughts and beliefs in response to a given situation. *A* stands for *antecedent event* (or trigger), *B* stands for *belief,* and *C* for *consequences.* I recently cared for a ninety-year-old man in the hospital who was also a brilliant clinical psychologist, and he explained *B* as "the bullshit you tell yourself." The ABC self-monitoring system makes abundantly clear how our own lens colors and refracts the world around us, and how there are consequences to our psychological overlay on reality. For example, imagine you are at a party with a group of people you know — from work, church, or another venue. At some point during the function, you look in the direction of one of these familiar faces and nod hello. Without appearing to respond to you, the person looks in another direction. *What is your first thought?*

If you're like many people, you think, "This person doesn't want to acknowledge me." Some people go a few steps further and decide, "This person doesn't want to acknowledge me because he is angry with me." Others leap still further, declaring, "Not only is this person angry with me, but I'm just not that likable, which is why I have trouble keeping friends." These automatic thoughts — which I liken to Tourette's syndrome tics of our inner dialogue — are often grossly distorted versions of what actually took place. Psychologists call them *cognitive distortions,* and they can be accompanied by some pretty unsavory feelings, ranging from mild uneasiness all the way to outright despair. In truth, you have no idea why the person didn't respond to you at the party. Maybe he was paying attention to what someone else was saying and didn't realize he even looked at you. Maybe he was trying to mentally process some other problem, and was just checked out. Maybe he *was* in fact angry with you — but you don't know that yet, and shouldn't assume it to be factual. Yet we do often take these automatic thoughts and the feelings that accompany them as if they were indisputable truths.

The ABC approach to cognitive distortions is to recognize them for what they are, and then actively replace them with more functional thoughts. First, name the *A*, the antecedent situation — in this case, your acquaintance failing to acknowledge your greeting. This may seem obvious, but it's important to parse out each component to clearly demonstrate to yourself that it's often not *only* the situation you're reacting to. Second, notice the *B*, beliefs, in response to the situation. These automatic thoughts are whatever your mind reflexively blurts out during your inner dialogue, and what my patient referred to as, ahem, baloney, because they can distort the truth in many ways. In this example, thinking that the person dissed you is an example of *jumping to conclusions.* Thinking that the reason behind the presumed diss is because that person is angry with you is an example of *personalization.* Believing that this one party incident proves you cannot maintain friendships is an example of *overgeneralization.* Certain outlooks, such as extreme pessimism, tend to involve a greater degree of cognitive distortion: "This didn't go well because I always screw things up." A related cognitive distortion is termed *filtering* — the tendency to filter out any positive aspects and focus relentlessly on the negative ones.

Incidentally, unrealistic optimism, which we discussed in chapter 2, happens when people inappropriately filter out all the negative, also distorting the truth.

The third step in ABC is to recognize the *C,* or consequences, of your automatic thoughts. At the very least, these consequences may make you feel uncomfortable. At worst, they may seriously hinder your friendships: If you are constantly leaping to assumptions about people, you're bound to be wrong at least some of the time, which can lead to divisive words or actions that drive wedges. But there are also consequences for your health and aging. Let's think back to the science lesson in chapter 1. Recall that our thoughts and feelings are literally carried throughout our bodies by the nervous, endocrine, immune, and cardiovascular systems (classic fight-or-flight responses), and leave their own biological footprints. Anxiety, self-doubt, and related thoughts and feelings are associated with increases in blood pressure, heart rate, and stress hormones such as adrenaline and cortisol, all of which pound our organs like waves on the beach. These thoughts and feelings may also erode our coping abilities and lead us toward harmful choices, as we saw with Joseph, who reached for a cigarette whenever he became stressed about his life situation, until he learned to preempt those anxious bouts with the new tools he learned in counseling, as well as with help from a nicotine patch. Whether we consider our stressors to be well founded and justifiable is irrelevant — if they are wearing us (and our telomeres) down to nubbins, we need to find new ways of handling them. Our outlook is key to this process.

There is a fourth step in the CBT process: Create an alternate way of looking at the situation by correcting the cognitive distortion. We could easily make this the *D* for *do-over* or *devise a new plan*. This step could be as simple as checking in with the other person involved in the situation and asking him directly. And we need to be open to the possibility that our acquaintance actually *is* miffed at us for some reason or another, and then cross that bridge if and when we come to it. Obviously, we don't need the ABC technique for every single negative thought racing through our heads. My rule of thumb is if something has crossed my mind more than five or so times in the same day, it's time to drop in, slow down my inner conversation, and take a closer look.

If you have never used CBT techniques

before, remember that this process will take practice to become as automatic as your current automatic thoughts. You are creating a new map for your thoughts and feelings.

Back when I first learned CBT techniques, I used a worksheet to write down the information for each of the four steps outlined here. While the steps make sense and seem easy enough to follow, I have found over time that I don't always acknowledge the distortion. Challenging one's own automatic thoughts is tough business! Sometimes even after acknowledging distortions, I don't always employ the discipline to correct them. This is where the help of a trained counselor or savvy confidant may be necessary.

Mindfulness

Mindfulness and CBT share a near-identical self-examination process. However, they differ in one fundamental way: *Mindfulness does not involve an attempt to change the content of the experience,* so you are not seeking to resolve cognitive distortions. Instead, mindfulness, as described by Dr. Jon Kabat-Zinn (founder of the Center for Mindfulness at the University of Massachusetts), refers to experiencing our thoughts, feelings, and physical sensations as they are in the here and now, without judging them and without actively trying to change them. Thus, when you mindfully drop in on your own inner dialogue, the quality of your self-examination is less judgmental because you are not labeling it as good, bad, distorted, or not distorted. When we are mindful, it is easier to recognize when our automatic thoughts are tending in a dangerous direction.

When I trained in the practice of mindfulness-based cognitive therapy, I was privileged to have one of the most esteemed teachers in the field, Dr. Zindel Segal, cognitive psychologist, researcher, academician, and coauthor with Mark Williams and John Teasdale of *Mindfulness Based Cognitive Therapy for Depression.* For people with a history of depression, Zindel referred to this negative spiraling of automatic thoughts as "entering the territory of depression" and described how mindfulness allowed people to remain alert so that they could, as soon as possible, read the signs (their own negative automatic thoughts) signaling entry into that dangerous territory and turn around. We do not have to have suffered from depression to employ these outlook GPS techniques, recognize when we're heading in an unhealthy direction, and maneuver ourselves accordingly. Next I'll show you how mindfully recognizing different mental "territories," or landscapes, works.

Not surprisingly, mindfulness has been especially effective in helping people with mental health conditions, such as by preventing relapse in depression, probably in large part because people learn to recognize the "territory" before they get too deep into it and can no longer adequately help themselves. More recent evidence from my colleagues Dr. David Wetter and Dr. Jennifer Vidrine, at the MD Anderson Cancer Center, suggests that mindfulness may also help prevent relapse to smoking (likely because people learn to recognize the "territory of relapse," which can be fraught with negative automatic thoughts and a strong craving).

Recall from chapter 1 that preliminary evidence suggests mindfulness may affect cellular processes such as telomere shortening. More research is needed in this arena, but there's no doubt that mindfulness practice offers a method to soften our fight-or-flight response to stressful situations — especially those in which this automatic response is not only not needed, but is actively detrimental. Depression, anxiety, and chronic pain are classic examples of chronic "whole body" stressors. Based on the research and my clinical experience, I believe that certain attitudes can be chronic whole body stressors, too. Over time, learning to blunt our own tendencies toward negative automatic responses may reduce overall wear and tear on our bodily organs.

How does mindfulness work in practice? Going back to the party example in which your acquaintance appeared to ignore you, steps 1 (A = antecedent event, or trigger) and 2 (B = belief, or BS you tell yourself) are identical to CBT. When it comes time for step 3 (C = consequences of our beliefs), we recognize the thought "I believed he didn't want to talk to me, because he was angry at me" for what it is — just a thought. We also notice any feelings that accompany that thought — "I felt sad that he didn't want to talk to me. I also felt embarrassed, because other people saw him snub me." Just being able to acknowledge our experience in this way often has the effect of lessening the emotional voltage of that experience. In mindfulness we also notice any associated physical sensations ("the pit in my stomach that arose when I believed he didn't want to talk to me"). This is called the *triangle of awareness,* in which we remain mentally centered in the midst of our thoughts, feelings, and physical sensations, each of which represents a point on the triangle. It's helpful to be on the lookout for all three of these aspects of experience, because they often travel in bundles.

To use a different example of a new and unproven business partner, the thought "I don't trust that person" may be accompanied by an anxious feeling, which is in turn accompanied by the sensation of queasiness. Occasionally, you may be able to pick up on only one aspect of this triad — the queasiness that turns out to be worry over mistrust of your business partner. Only later may you recognize how the queasiness relates to uncomfortable thoughts and feelings about this person.

Mindfulness does not have a correlate to step four of the CBT process, which is actively trying to stamp out our cognitive distortions as soon as we recognize them. Practicing mindfulness, we are not trying to correct, change, or replace our experience *in this moment.* We simply experience it for what it is, with a little more perspective than we had before, so that our future actions are based on greater awareness (and a less distorted version) of any given situation. Practicing mindfulness, like practicing CBT, helps us become more aware of our own mental traffic and inner conversation and can allow us to gain a little distance from it. And the more mindful we are, the better our awareness of our own traits and how we might want to change them. Mindfulness is simply choosing to be aware of whatever you are thinking, feeling, and sensing *right now.* If you feel tingling excitement in your chest, your attention moves there. The same goes even for less positive thoughts and feelings: If you feel pain in your left big toe, you let your attention rest on that pain, as opposed to actively trying to ease the pain. When you learn to confront the gamut of your experience without getting too riled, your mind and body benefit.

To help you better understand how mindfulness can benefit you in a real-world context, I've pulled an example from my own research with Drs. Golnaz Tabibnia, David Creswell, Hedy Kober, and Cecilia Westbrook and colleagues. In this study, we showed visual cues (pictures) of cigarettes to men and women who were trying to quit smoking. We then asked them about their experience of craving and measured their brain activity in response to the cues using fMRI. The same men and women were asked to view the visual cues under a few different conditions. We termed one of these conditions *mindful attending,* in which the participants were given instructions to "notice and accept" any experience brought on by the cues. We termed another condition *passive looking,* meaning participants were to view the pictures similar to the way they might watch TV or a movie. We found that during mindful attending to a cigarette cue, as compared to passively looking, people reported lower levels of craving *and* had lower neural activation in craving-specific areas of the brain such as the anterior cingulate cortex (ACC). Other research shows that lower levels of craving do actually translate into smoking fewer cigarettes. (In our study, we did not offer the men and women the opportunity to smoke after the experiment, which would have been an unfair temptation for people who were trying to quit smoking.)

In his poem "The Guest House," the thirteenth-century poet Jalaluddin Rumi likens each of us to a guesthouse, and our thoughts and feelings to unexpected visitors. He urges us to "Welcome and entertain them all!" Tying this to the preceding example, a craving is one of these visitors: often unexpected and usually unwelcome when one is grappling with trying to change one's behavior toward drugs, food, sex —

you name it. When you are practicing mindfulness, just as when you are practicing any of the self-examination techniques, you're getting to know these guests before you send them on their way. The act of "sitting with them" (mindfully attending) in and of itself seems to alter our emotional and cognitive reactivity toward them, which over time may translate into fewer episodes in which our fight-or-flight system is activated. This, in turn, means less wear and tear on our bodies as well as better decision making (i.e., we don't cave to the cigarette or the chocolate cake). Mindfulness is the very antithesis of suppression, which most psychologists agree is a losing strategy: Try to slam the door on these "unexpected visitors" and they will only knock louder.

I want to stress that being mindful does not make you an automaton. We can ride our emotional waves, but remain just slightly separate from them, and in doing so, maintain some control over their awesome power. The late Alan Marlatt coined the term *urge surfing* to characterize this process for craving. (But you could just as easily substitute "anger surfing" or "sadness surfing" to describe mindfully attending to the feeling-waves that propagate through us moment by moment.) It's thought that this ability to detach ever so slightly from our thoughts and feelings is one of the key ways in which mindfulness helps us avoid relapse, by cultivating what Franciscan priest and social activist Richard Rohr refers to as *emotional sobriety,* a state of healthy separation from our inner conversation that we can achieve via several routes, including CBT, mindfulness, and contemplation.

Contemplation

Contemplation is a practice that may be especially comforting to people for whom spirituality is important. Of course, spirituality does not need to be tied to God, per se, and this can be a very helpful technique even for agnostic and some atheist outlook travelers. Also called contemplative prayer, contemplation harks back to an early Christian tradition very similar to mindfulness. In contemplation, a person enters what Richard Rohr and other teachers refer to as an "inner room," the sanctuary in which the mind is free from judgment and dualistic thinking — good/bad, black/white, right/ wrong, etc. Incidentally, this all-or-nothing dualism is recognized in CBT as a cognitive distortion called *polarized thinking* — you're either perfect or perfectly horrible. Yet in contemplation, as in mindfulness, the practitioner is not trying to actively stamp out the cognitive distortions so much as to simply notice his or her own thoughts and feelings. The actual process of mindfulness and contemplation is essentially identical, so that all of the explanations I've provided for mindfulness, and how it may ultimately help us to reduce some of our own harmful reactivity, apply here as well.

The main difference between mindfulness and contemplation is that at its core, contemplation is a practice in which the contemplator seeks to come closer to a higher spiritual power. The process is explained most clearly by Father Thomas Keating, an abbot and one of three founders of *centering prayer,* a contemporary version of contemplation based on the fourteenth-century anonymous English text *The Cloud of Unknowing.* During centering prayer, the main intention is to establish and maintain union with God. In his book *Intimacy with God: An Introduction to Centering Prayer,* Father Keating describes the process as the intention to "consent to God's presence and action during the time of prayer." Together, Fathers Keating and Rohr have taught contemplation and centering prayer to thousands, helping them cultivate emotional sobriety.

Anyone who has had the experience of being completely swept away by negative emotions (that means you and me both) understands that emotional sobriety is a welcome refuge for anyone, including card-carrying atheists. When we are emotionally sober we remain alive to our own experiences, but do not become intoxicated by them, which, as you now understand, activates your stress response systems and can lead you to make poor choices for your health and aging. As an example of stress intoxication, let's say you are highly distressed over an ongoing rivalry with a coworker. You come home after one particularly difficult day and stew about this in your kitchen. During this time your body is preparing for battle: Your breathing, heart rate, and blood pressure rise, your muscles become tense, even your platelets become "stickier" as they prepare to clot your blood — an evolutionary response to help prevent you from bleeding to death if you are gored by an animal tusk, spear, or other sharp object that threatened our ancestors. Within minutes you've consumed twelve chocolate chip cookies, half a bag of potato chips, three beers — you fill in the blank — and are now nauseated and sluggish for the rest of the evening. Sound familiar?

Now contrast that with a contemplative approach to the same situation. You may still feel distressed about the coworker situation, but this time you take a detour from the usual stress highway to fight-or-flight. You walk into your home and sit down for a moment to consciously acknowledge your distress, recognizing that the thoughts and feelings you are experiencing right now are just that — thoughts and feelings; they are not *you.* They will pass. Taking this time to breathe — literally and figuratively — calms your body and clears your mind by reorienting you before you react. (You may first need to get on a treadmill or run around the block a few times to clear your head — if that's the case, go for it.) Perhaps you need to set up a meeting with the coworker and hash things out. Perhaps you realize that the coworker has very little to do with your state of mind, but ironically, has pointed to something about yourself that you'd like to work on (maybe you realize you're too possessive, or that you need to boost your self-esteem so that other people's opinions don't bother you as much). Whatever realizations arise during this moment of contemplation, acknowledge them.

Note that contemplative practice, just like the other techniques we're discussing, does not necessarily mean that you instantly feel better. Rather, it means that you remain "sober" enough to see your way to the next step, which may be to exercise or to ask for spiritual help, or identify another way to safely metabolize your tension. In the end you may still decide to eat some of the chips and cookies, or drink a beer, but you are doing so with full awareness, which helps you make better decisions (i.e., consuming less).

Years before I met Richard Rohr, my mother taught me what has become the focal point of my own contemplative practice. One day during a crisis she reminded me that in any situation, there are solutions, even if I couldn't see them at the moment. The first step in cultivating emotional sobriety is recognizing this fact. The second step is asking for help, which can take many forms. Through contemplation, you are giving yourself the opportunity to ask for spiritual and material help — whether it comes from within or without — to recognize and embrace these solutions.

While centering prayer is a viable path to emotional sobriety, it is not the only path. Emotional sobriety is a destination, whether we arrive there through CBT, mindfulness, contemplation/centering prayer, following "typical doctor advice" (as I'll discuss in the next chapter), or some other means. When we understand how a strongly negative outlook engenders negative emotional states that leave their footprints on our biology, it's easier to see how valuable emotional sobriety is for our own health and aging.

Guided Imagery

Guided imagery is a mind-body therapy that involves voluntarily thinking about specific mental images — usually in combination with progressive muscle relaxation and deep breathing — to improve health. It has been successfully used in clinical settings (such as the interventional radiology suite, where many medical procedures are performed) to reduce stress, anxiety, and pain. Guided imagery is another method for tuning in to our inner conversation, and here we're using our imagination as the primary tool. Of all the techniques I've introduced so far, this one is, in my opinion, the most fun to work with. The term *imagery* is a bit of a misnomer in that it refers to any of our senses that help us to imagine, not just the visual. We recruit our sense of hearing, taste, smell, touch, sight, and any combination thereof to allow an image to form in our minds of whatever we'd like to explore. Images are a natural language for many of us.

If we can briefly slow down our internal dialogue long enough to take a look at it, we gain yet another window into our current outlook in action and catch glimpses of a new outlook. We can also use guided imagery to become more familiar with our thoughts and feelings the way Rumi encourages us to greet them like visitors in a guesthouse. Much like viewing online photos of our next vacation spot, we can use imagery to evoke excitement and strengthen our volition to reach future goals. In one of my smoking cessation classes, one middle-aged woman told me after the first exercise that her self-image was of a frail, hunched lady sitting on her porch. Over the course of six guided imagery sessions, she cultivated a vision of herself standing upright, taking deep, regular breaths, and feeling warm sun on her face. She used this second image frequently to remind herself of the nonsmoker she wanted to become.

To get your brain thinking along these lines, first try imagining the taste of jelly. (This exercise actually appears on one of the psychological scales to help a person assess his or her ability to imagine.) Your brain instantly recruits the memory of your last jelly encounter, replete with all the sensory information from that experience, and conjures the taste. You may have recently eaten grape jelly on white toast, or you may have tried a fancy habanero-mango jelly on grilled salmon. Whatever the details, your brain fills them in — you can easily bring to mind sounds, touch, and other senses. Once you get the hang of it, you can try imagery with an eye toward change. Let's say you want to start exercising again but can't seem to muster the volition to do so. Imagine the last time you were in (better) shape — even if it was when you were fourteen; it still counts! How did you feel physically? Emotionally? What sorts of clothes were you wearing during this period of your life? What types of fun things were you doing, and whom were you hanging out with? As you bring to mind all of these details of yourself during that time, imagine yourself doing some type of physical activity — running, swimming, dancing, jumping rope, whatever you want to be doing — and tell yourself you can start to do this *now*. We can "dose" ourselves with these motivating images, using them to guide ourselves into a new reality.

Athletes use visualization to hone their attitudes *and* their technique. In fact, one of my very first guided imagery "teachers" was Eric Soderholm, former third baseman for the Chicago White Sox, who taught me how to bat when I was a timid fourteen-year-old high school student. I had decent natural coordination, but my head position was undisciplined. Like many hitters, I lacked confidence at the plate and often looked up prematurely to see where the ball would go, which meant I took my eyes off of it before making contact with my bat, resulting in a lot of big fat strikes. As a consequence of these two problems, I didn't make the softball team my freshman year of high school. Devastated, I moped around the house for two weeks, until my mom (always in the know) discovered that Mr. Soderholm, who had retired from professional baseball due to a knee injury, not only was a resident of our town but also offered coaching sessions.

Eric gave me tips through a series of three lessons, the last of which ended in "PMA" — his shorthand for "positive mental attitude." The first couple of lessons involved exactly what I expected to learn from a pro — expert technical instruction for body positioning and timing. The PMA was something entirely different. Eric sat me down in a big comfy chair situated in the middle of what looked like a mini recording studio. He gave me a pair of headphones and then walked into a separate room and began speaking into a microphone. I remember closing my eyes and hearing his confident, animated voice through the headphones, encouraging me to imagine myself at bat, watching the pitcher wind up and release, cocking my hips one tiny bit clockwise to give that extra "bam" of power into my swing, and looking straight down the barrel of the bat until the moment of contact. Then as I was really getting into the exercise, he planted a seed that has stuck with me to this day: "It doesn't matter if God is up on the mound — you hit that ball." I immediately took the suggestion and visualized a fastball pitched by God Almighty Himself. And I swung. And I hit it! Later, on the field, I recalled this image every time I went to bat. The next year, I made the team as the designated hitter.

Similar to CBT, mindfulness, and contemplation, guided imagery can be led by a trained counselor or health care provider, but there are also CDs and downloadables that you can use at home. (See Resources at the end of the book for suggestions for commercially available audio scripts.) To help you learn the basics, I've included an actual script of guided imagery that I used in my own studies. The first research project I undertook during my training at Harvard was a clinical trial of guided imagery to help people quit smoking. This study featured a specific interactive style of guided imagery developed by David Bresler, Ph.D., and Martin Rossman, M.D., who together had founded the Academy for Guided Imagery to train health professionals in this practice. David and Marty are two phenomenal outlook guides, each with his own approach to mind-body medicine. David is the author of *Free Yourself from Pain,* while Marty has written *Guided Imagery for Self-Healing, Fighting Cancer from Within,* and *The Worry Solution.*

I continue to recommend their techniques to patients, friends, neighbors, and family, and I regularly use them myself. While guided imagery in general is a powerful (and fun!) mind-body therapy, Interactive Guided Imagery, which David and Marty developed, lets our imaginations do the walking and talking, and avoids scripting our experience for us. I'll show you an example in a moment.

In my study, I tested the short-term (six- and twelve-week) and long-term (one year) quit rates of people who went through the

Interactive Guided Imagery program. I also trained in guided imagery so that I could deliver the treatment to the men and women participating in the trial. When I began my study, I gave the participants a CD and workbook to take home, which Marty and David had designed and recorded specifically for the study, and each week for six weeks my subjects came to a group guided-imagery class led by yours truly. The first two lessons introduced total body relaxation and taught participants to access an inner safe place — a venue, either real or imagined, in which they felt safe and powerful, a place filled with infinite possibility. The third lesson encouraged them to formulate an action plan for quitting smoking, by setting specific goals and rehearsing (imagining) successful completion of those goals. They then practiced refining their action plans through several additional imagery exercises, including envisioning themselves as a nonsmoker, recalling positive past events, and devising ways to increase positive activities in their current lives.

The fourth lesson involved meeting an inner adviser, which could be someone (a relative) or something (a favorite animal) they knew in real life, or someone or something imagined. (Remember, this is the world of imagination!) The only criteria for an inner adviser was that it needed to be both wise and fully in the participant's corner. The purpose of the adviser was to boost confidence and motivation. In the fifth lesson, study participants imagined their own resistance to quitting smoking — the parts of them that really wanted to continue smoking. Anyone who has made behavior change understands that we first must acknowledge our inner conflicts before we can resolve them: Sometimes we desperately want to do the very things that we desperately want to *stop* doing. Finally, people rehearsed a plan in the very probable event that they relapsed (relapse occurs in up to nine out of ten unaided quit attempts, and most relapse happens within the first week).

Without question, everyone's favorite exercise was "Meeting Your Ideal Self." This exercise, like all of them, began with instructions for relaxation and deep breathing, and is very similar to the scripted guided imagery that you will find on a CD, or even during a session with a counselor. Here are verbal instructions I used for my trial participants during group classes: *When you're ready, close your eyes and focus on your breathing. Let your body breathe accord-*

ing to its own natural rhythm. You may want to imagine a ball of energy or white light that starts at your lower abdomen and rises to your forehead each time you inhale. As you exhale, the energy descends along your spine, down your legs, and into the ground.

The exercise soon became more open-ended, inviting the participants to let their imaginations creatively fill in the space. Because this was a study to help people quit smoking cigarettes, the content was tobacco-specific: *As you focus on your breathing, think about how good it would feel if you really were able to break the smoking habit once and for all. What would it be like to have no desires or urges to smoke? Now allow an image to form of yourself as a successful nonsmoker.*

Finally, we used sensory recruitment (i.e., engaging all of the five senses) to bring the image alive: *Imagine looking exactly the way you'd want to look, and feeling exactly the way you'd like to feel after you've quit for good. Notice every detail about yourself — what you're wearing, the expression on your face, your posture. Notice how confident you are . . . how much energy you have . . . how easily you can breathe . . . and move. . . . Notice how good it feels to experience yourself this way.*

While this particular script was designed for people who were trying to quit smoking, the take-home point for you, whether you smoke or not, is the *process*. In a relaxed state, you fully call to mind an image, and then use that image to assist you in the process of improving your health. Sometimes the image enhances your insights about beliefs that may be holding you back. Other times, the imagery directly motivates you to take action toward better health. Using guided imagery, we not only pay attention to our thoughts, feelings, and physical sensations — the triangle of awareness we learned about in mindfulness — but we take the process a step further by giving our outlook a "face." We can even learn to cultivate different aspects of this face, or envision a new one altogether, in the service of healthy aging.

Motivational Interviewing

Motivational interviewing, or MI, is a process that was developed by psychologists Dr. William Miller and Dr. Stephen Rollnick, and is essentially a style of conversation designed to help a person realize his or her true goals and act in line with those aspirations. For example, if one of your long-term goals is to be able to be physically fit enough to run after your grand-children, yet you are not doing any kind of exercise and continue to put on weight, then you are by definition actively working against your own plan. You know what you want to do. The big question is, how do you get there?

MI helps answer that question. It's a tool that helps the road open up before you. MI shows you how to see the path and gives you a starting push in the right direction. It is typically conducted by a health professional, but in this exercise you're interviewing yourself, and it can be just as effective solo if you practice it regularly. There are four basic principles of motivational interviewing: 1) expressing empathy, 2) developing discrepancy, 3) rolling with resistance, and 4) supporting self-efficacy. Expressing empathy simply means putting yourself in another person's shoes: "Losing weight and toning up takes work — I understand what you're up against." It's quite possible to put yourself in your own shoes, so to speak, by thinking about yourself as a friend you'd be talking to. Acknowledging the difficult road ahead with empathy for yourself is the first and most critical of the MI steps, because it allows you to become and remain your own ally. As we all know by now, we are sometimes our own worst enemy, and as you listen more intently to your inner conversation, you may be shocked at just how harsh the inner critic can be (more on self-compassion in chapter 6). When it comes to attitudinal change, you are much more helpful to yourself as an ally than as a critic.

The second MI tool, developing discrepancy, is simply acknowledging any gaps between what you are currently doing and what you want to be doing. Going back to the previous example, obesity and lack of physical fitness both take you in the exact opposite direction of the youthfulness you desire to keep up with your grandchild. Whatever your unique situation, you must be willing to see where change is needed. But change can be hard and our own resistance to change can be fierce. So as you learn to examine your inner conversation, listen for the *resistance talk* and take the third step of motivational interviewing: Roll with it! Resistance talk is essentially whatever your mind comes up with in defense of the status quo. Staying with our example, resistance talk may sound something like, "Oh, I don't really need to keep up my dietary and fitness plan — I can walk just as fast as other people my own age." (The problem is, if the people with whom you are comparing yourself are also overweight and physically unfit, you need a new point of reference!) Resistance to change may be so tenacious that you maintain your position even in the face of strong evidence to the contrary — for example, despite your own panting after running or walking up a flight of stairs.

And lest you think I'm getting too high on my horse, I confess that until very recently I was in full-blown denial about my waning exercise capacity, primarily because I hadn't challenged myself physically for a couple of years. Driving to and from work and taking elevators everywhere, I didn't realize how deconditioned I had become. I even thought (erroneously) that because I could walk briskly up Cardiac Hill on the University of Pittsburgh campus — so named for its steepness, which according to local lore has precipitated more than a few heart attacks — that I was still in decent shape. Then one day at a park I found myself in a game of tag with my children, and I couldn't catch them! I remained "it" for almost a half hour, and finally gave up — in between desperate heaves trying to catch my breath. I was only forty-one at the time, and I had no choice but to hear my own resistance talk and admit that I needed an exercise plan. If I didn't take action now, I would not be playing any tag in the coming years. So I told myself exactly what I tell my patients: "If you want to be a healthy fiftysomething, you need to start by being a healthy fortysomething." (Fill in the blanks depending on your own age.) However "young" you want to be when you're "old," start living that way *now*.

The "roll with resistance" concept was originally designed to sidestep the antagonism that often develops when the health care provider advocates one direction — "You need to lose weight" — and the patient or client resists, either outwardly or inwardly: "No I won't, and you can't make me!" Make a pact with yourself to stay honest, learn to hear your own resistance talk, recognize it for what it is, and roll with it. This is key to outlook and behavior change, and in principle it's really no different than the techniques we've already reviewed. While you are rolling with resistance, listen for the *change talk*. Change talk is whatever parts of your inner conversation favor change: "It would really be nice if I weren't spending seventy-five dollars every weekend getting smashed," or "Boy, would I love to look hot in a pair of shorts." These are the thoughts and feelings that intuitively propel you forward, and they also help you maintain your position once you've gained some attitudinal ground. Learning to recognize and act on change talk is the primary goal of this technique.

So where do you get the gumption to act on your change talk? This is where the fourth step of motivational interviewing, supporting self-efficacy, comes in. Self-efficacy, or self-support, is your belief in your ability to succeed, regardless of how small or large that success may be. In a sense you become your own cheerleader, and you can adjust the dose of rah-rah up or down as you see fit. Even if you don't have a lot of self-efficacy to start with, there are ways to bolster yourself, with two particularly powerful techniques.

The first is called *looking back,* which is mining your memory banks to find examples from your own experience in which you were able to accomplish something, even if it was long ago. For example, if you want to begin eating healthier, and there was a period, however brief or however long ago, during which you successfully ate for the benefit of your body, bring that time and situation to mind now. Be careful not to brush off your accomplishments because you deem them to be too small or too short-lived — there is no such thing. To extract maximum motivation and propel yourself forward *now,* you'll want to remember all of the details while you look back (and in doing so, you are practicing guided imagery). In addition to helping you build on the successes of the past, looking back can also be a very powerful technique to learn where things may have gone wrong, and figure out ways to avoid those pitfalls in the future. Maybe you took a new job with longer hours and let nutrition fall by the wayside — how might you prioritize healthy eating once again?

The second major tool to boost your self-efficacy is *looking forward,* in which you imagine a scene that has not yet come to pass. You can start with a past success and embellish by recruiting all of your senses, similar to the previous guided imagery exercise, and then make it up as you go along — after all, you are imagining! For example, I envision myself years down the road, taking a hike with my (now older) daughters and dogs along the Columbia River Gorge, hearing their laughter over the booming mist of Multnomah Falls. When you can envision the future in this way, you can aim your brain toward a clear target, and stand a greater chance of getting there.

Incidentally, looking forward is a technique that optimists tend to do well. Recall when I described in the first chapter the neuroimaging research showing that when optimists, as compared to pessimists, imagined future positive events, their brains were more active during the exercise. But whatever our attitude latitude, we can learn to employ these techniques to help ourselves.

Outlook Examination Tools: Recap

To review, we've covered five practices: cognitive behavioral therapy (CBT), mindfulness, contemplative prayer/contemplation, guided imagery, and motivational interviewing. Use one or all of these five practices to home in on the unique details of your outlook terrain — its hills, valleys, and weather patterns. These techniques help us go beyond the scales we completed in step 1 (determining our current attitude latitude, or Point A) and probe other, less well-traveled territories of our character, such as our deepest motivations and fears, which are tough to elicit from a questionnaire. The ability to eavesdrop on and change our inner conversation doesn't necessarily come easily for all of us, including me, and we need to learn and practice these listening skills. Even if we do pay close attention, we may do so in ways that are not entirely beneficial. That is, we may judge ourselves and others harshly, or get stuck on repeat cycles of negative thoughts that turn out to be a lot less productive than we may think they are. So you can see how paying attention is a complex process, and one that requires practice and guidance. For each of these techniques in step 3, it is helpful to first get comfortable and practice them before moving on to further steps for concrete attitudinal change, which I discuss in the next chapter.

My Own Path to Outlook Change

So what does the step-by-step journey of outlook change look like in an actual person? Let's go down my own memory lane to get a clearer picture of the process. Several years ago, when I first started studying how optimism and cynical hostility predict cardiovascular disease and death among women, I completed step 1 and determined my attitude latitude without any conscious desire to change. While I had been fascinated by the mind-body connection for many years, I had been more focused on the outlook of my patients and research participants, and had not stopped to fully consider my own coordinates. I remember that my first reaction on seeing these results was one of surprise: *"Me, pessimistic?!"* (That was an overreaction, as I'm not actually highly pessimistic. I just didn't score as highly optimistic as I thought I would.) As the results of my research study continued to unfold, eventually showing that the most optimistic women, compared with the most pessimistic, had a lower risk of heart attack and death, and that the most cynical women, compared with the least cynical, had a higher risk of death, I could not help but wonder how they might apply to me. Just like you, I wanted to stack the aging deck in my favor.

While the research participants in my study were much older than I was, the links between outlook and physical health have been made across all age groups, from elementary school through retirement. So my relatively young age didn't give me a get-out-of-jail-free card. I knew that certain aspects of my outlook weren't on the firmest footing, yet I didn't think to try and do anything about it at first. I walked around for a couple of years with this knowledge gnawing at me. Despite this nagging discomfort, it took me months to move on to step 2 and formulate an intention to change.

I did, however, start paying more attention to other people's outlooks, and I knew several good friends and family members well enough to get some close-up, candid shots. Fortunately for me, my husband is one of the most optimistic people I know; I'd say he's right up there with Leon Varley from chapter 2. While I wasn't necessarily aiming my own brain in any particular direction yet, I did watch how he aimed his. As I witnessed his optimism in action, I became increasingly enamored of the process and wanted more — kind of like the café scene in *When Harry Met Sally,* when the woman (the late Estelle Reiner) at a nearby table witnesses Sally's (Meg Ryan) ecstasy and deadpans to her waiter, "I'll have what she's having." This desire to rewire served as the impetus for step 2, aiming my own brain in the desired direction to greater optimism — my own Point B.

I remember walking back from a lunch break one day and listening to my husband, who is also a physician and researcher, enthusiastically describe a new research project. In the course of five minutes he outlined all of the necessary steps for this study of people living with HIV — designing, funding, implementing it, and publishing and disseminating the results to make them available to the people who needed them. He had a plan for how to use the momentum gained at each stage to get to the next stage — sort of like artfully bounding one's way through an obstacle course.

"So how do you *know* this part will work as planned?" I asked, fixated on the need for certainty. More than a few of us still cling to a need to have things totally worked out before we can optimistically embrace a plan or project. But of course, that is not what dispositional optimism is all about. Dispositional optimism is expecting a bright future *in the face of uncertainty.* My husband fully understood that not every step would work out as planned, but he was certain that he could mobilize the resources to figure out a reasonable solution when the time came.

The most striking thing I observed about his process was that he often viewed his goals as if they had already happened. This occurred to me one day when he used the past tense to describe a future event (a habit of his that I had long found grammatically irritating and temporally confusing). Once I realized the amazing process that was taking shape in his mind, my irritation ceased. He really did see the end result, and he knew he could create it — so much so that he spoke about it as if he already had! While he wouldn't have labeled it as such, he naturally employed the motivational interviewing technique of looking forward, which, as we have seen, deploys the imagination through a form of guided imagery.

During this and other opportunities to see other people's outlook in action, I compared them with my own process, and wondered what it would be like if I could learn to visualize the finished product more of the time, and borrow the momentum of that inner experience to create the outer experience. Depending on the situation, the visualized product may in fact be each step in the process that gets you to the next step, or it could be the grand finale itself. Fortunately, during this time I also had the benefit of regularly teaching mindfulness, guided imagery, CBT, and other techniques for outlook cultivation, such as self-compassion — all of which not only afforded me some mandatory practice time but also gave me hundreds of practice partners. Like many clinicians and investigators, I have learned a ton from patients and research participants.

Each time I did these exercises, I became more and more interested in step 3: examining my outlook in action, by paying attention to my own thoughts and feelings as they arose. Although I had been practicing these exercises for years, they took on greater relevance under my developing hypothesis that outlook is a driver of biological aging, and I became more invested. Sometimes we really do need a carrot to help focus and strengthen our intention, and the sooner you identify yours, whether it is healthy aging or some other incentive, the more likely you are to begin walking the steps to attitudinal change.

Fueled by my own curiosity about the link between outlook and aging, I found it easier to focus on the positive and let go of a greater proportion of the negative when I examined my thoughts and feelings. Recall that what I'm referring to as negative aspects are the often supercharged, automatic thoughts that pop up from moment to moment. Some of us may have fewer negative pop-ups than others, but we all have them. Over a number of months, I told myself more and more regularly that I not only wanted to but was also *able* to alter some of this inner talk. At some point, I made the intention to try to approach situations a little more optimistically, and to approach people with less cynicism. After a while, this conscious exercise became part of my routine, and I even started posting the reminder stickies in my car and office, as I told you earlier. Over several years, these baby steps constituted the fundamentals of my attitudinal travel. Mind you, I was not striving for huge change; making these non-ambitious outlook travel plans kept the process fun and the benchmark attainable. But I do wish someone had laid out these steps for me, because I believe that they catalyze the process of cultivating a healthier outlook.

If you are still uncertain of how you might walk steps 1 through 3 in the service of your own outlook, my recommendation is this: *Pretend!* Choose one aspect of your outlook that you're not too hot on or curious about tweaking, and for just a moment, imagine what it would be like to change this facet. As I related in my softball example, the pathway to designated hitter began by cultivating a can-do attitude. Along the lines of "what if," sometimes we can learn the most about our own struggles by relating to the struggles of fictional characters — one of the great healing properties of story.

One night I was sitting on the couch with my kids watching the third Harry Potter movie, *The Prisoner of Azkaban,* when I made an extraordinary realization. In this story, Harry Potter illustrates optimism in action by combining intention, guided imagery, motivational interviewing, and, of course, a dose of magic. This may sound like a stretch, but the scene I'm about to describe illustrates the definition of optimism that I offered you in the first chapter: the ability to visualize your own bright future as real, and bring it to the present moment.

For those of you who aren't familiar with Harry Potter, he is a down-on-his-luck orphan who, by his own talent, hard work, help from others, and fate, has become the rising star wizard of the magic world. In this scene, Harry is standing at the edge of a pond with his injured godfather and only living relative, Sirius Black, when the pair are suddenly attacked by dementors, destructive ghosts who have come to capture Sirius.

In Harry's world, the only known defense against a dementor is the Expecto Patronum spell (translated as "I desire a protector"). The spell activates a body of light representing one's deepest, most positive feelings, and literally brings hope alive in the form of whatever the person casting the spell imagines — in Harry's case, a stag. Harry attempts the spell, but doubts his own abilities and is soon overpowered by a swarm of dementors. He has a vision of a figure with a stag beating back the dementors on the opposite shore, and is then magically transported a few moments in time to find himself back in mortal danger, although this time from the vantage point of the valiant figure on the opposite bank that he had seen moments earlier. Once he realizes that the apparition was actually *him,* he is able to conjure a brilliant stag and defeat the dementors. In psychological terms, Harry was able to look forward, and from that vantage point look back in time to envision his ideal self, from which hope emanated so invincibly that it literally saved his life.

The process of watching and cultivating one's outlook in this way *is* magical, but it does not only live in the mind of J. K. Rowling. It is well within the reach of even the densest muggle (Harry Potter–speak for non-magic folk like you and me). Imagine what it would be like if you could live every moment, or even just one moment, this way! Think of one situation and imagine, just like you used to do when you were a child. What if you knew deep down that you could see that situation to a good resolution? How would things be different? How much anxiety and fear would that sense of certainty wash away? What would that absence of distress then allow you to accomplish? Pick one thing in your life, however small, and start approaching it this way. Once you can do it one time, you can do it again. And again.

5
THE SAVVY OUTLOOK
TRAVELER 3:
STAYING ON TRACK

Now that we've reviewed how steps 1, 2, and 3 help people move *up,* we're ready to discuss some additional footwork for outlook change. I think of these as stabilizer steps to keep you on a good path once you've already started, although some people may actually *begin* their outlook journey as they encounter these guideposts. As I've stressed before, there are many onramps along the road to outlook change. You'll find that these steps are as much a key to healthy aging as they are to attitudinal change, underscoring how intertwined our outlook is with our health. The idea is to get ourselves aligned — to get the mind and body working together toward the goal of healthy aging. You do not need to follow the steps in any particular order, or follow each step perfectly. As you read, notice what you are drawn to and begin there. Move at whatever speed you're able to handle. Then as you get going, you can kick it into higher gear.

STEP 4: ACKNOWLEDGE YOUR ACCOMPLISHMENTS ALONG THE WAY

Giving yourself credit for meeting a goal is more than just a superficial nod. It actually highlights the accomplishment as concrete evidence that you really *can* make changes. The easiest way to create that evidence in the first place is to set a truly attainable goal, which may mean starting small. For example, if your weight has yo-yoed before and the very thought of resolving to lose twenty pounds results in heart palpitations, break up your goal into bite-size pieces to make it less daunting and more likely that you'll succeed in hitting your target. Instead of thinking about the task in aggregate ("I have to work out for at least three hours a week!"), think of it in small doses ("I'll walk thirty minutes a day during lunch."). I do this, and I also huff and puff my way up six flights of stairs to my office a couple of times a day. Then — and this is critical — reflect on your accomplishment, even if it seems insignificant or silly: "I climbed six flights of stairs," or "I walked for five minutes." Now, who says you can't do it again? Acknowledging your success in this way arms you with data to challenge those "I can't" notions with concrete, irrefutable evidence that you *can*.

I can't underscore the importance of this step enough. I myself have to regularly call my attention back to my abilities (via sticky notes, iPhone alerts, and frequent pep talks from my husband and friends that start with "Remember, you can do this") in order to avoid the tendency to fixate on what I *haven't* done, and keep building. Instead, we must recognize the accomplishments that it took to make it this far, and spell out the achievable steps to reach a desired goal. Kids need to learn to acknowledge their successes at an early age, because it helps them avoid undue frustration and spend their energies pursuing the activities they love. Such pursuits keep us younger as we grow older, regardless of our age.

Recently, I watched this process develop in my own six-year-old daughter during her first tennis lesson. She was excited to be there and was raring to hit the ball. Her instructor, who was also the coach of the local high school girls' and boys' teams and an expert motivator, made a game of trying to get to ten continuous rallies. My daughter *really* wanted to get to ten, but in the first few minutes was only reaching four or five.

She kept running off the court to bury her head in my husband's newspaper, despondent, and each time we had to coax her back to the lesson. Over the course of the next half hour, she was able to rally to eight, but instead of focusing on the thrill of her rapid improvement, she remained fixated on what she perceived as her failure to get to ten. At one point she dragged her racket on the ground and declared that she didn't like tennis and didn't want to come back.

Her coach, who had seen this all before, didn't bat an eye. He kept tossing balls over the net, pointing out several facts, including "It's hard to get to ten" and "Not many people get to ten when they first start out." When she reached nine, my daughter still had a pout on her face, prompting him to tell her, "That's one more than you did before — you can't be unhappy with nine." By the end of the lesson, she had surpassed ten and reached thirteen rallies. As we all clapped and cheered, her coach gave her a high five, leaned over the net, and said, "You just learned a really important lesson and you're going to need this for tennis. Anytime you're trying to do something and you can't quite get it, what do you need to remember?" Her little face looked up at him and she nodded earnestly as he told her, "You need to keep trying."

Be honest — how many times have you slumped around the proverbial tennis court and wanted to give up? Obviously, you don't need to play tennis to glean the message from this lesson. My daughter might have given up had her coach (and her parents) not urged her to acknowledge each small step of success, one rally at a time. Acknowledging our accomplishments helps stop our negative spirals in their tracks, while simultaneously stoking our enthusiasm to continue on to greater feats. Several months later, my little girl was following her desire to hit the ball fifty times, and had made it up to thirty-seven. How different would your life be if you could block out more of the "I can't" messages and remember the "keep trying" messages sooner in the game?

Learning to recognize the unique way the "I can't" messages manifest for each one of us — and how we can block those thoughts when they surface — naturally lifts us up to higher ground, providing a new vantage point from which we can clearly see even more outlook guideposts. Over the years, what I have found most surprising in my medical practice is just how often people allow largely erroneous "I can't" beliefs to define their health and set the pace for their aging. Whether we overeat, underexercise, smoke, or persist in abusive personal and professional relationships, somewhere along the way these "I can't" messages often seep in and take hold: "I've already had a heart attack, so weight loss doesn't matter now," or "Every time I try to stop smoking I get so bitchy, my family tells me to start again," and my favorite, "I have to die of *something.*"

The latter statement is actually a form of "I can't," because it essentially assumes that whatever you're doing now will proceed unchecked until death. It is certain that we will all die. But there is no rule that says you have to age at light speed, be debilitated and sickened on your way to your grave, or die earlier than the fates intended. I've already discussed how unhealthy behaviors, including smoking, hazardous drinking, eating unhealthy food, and lack of exercise are associated with getting older before our time by predisposing us to heart attacks, cancer, stroke, and other debilitating diseases. There is mounting evidence that these health behaviors are associated with older age on a cellular level. I coauthored a study with my colleagues Dr. Yan Song, Dr. Simin Liu, and others on how these health behaviors affect our telomeres — those "protective shoelace tips" on the ends of our DNA, which are barometers of cellular wear and tear. People with lower lifestyle scores — meaning they exhibited generally poorer health behaviors — had shorter telomeres compared with those with a better lifestyle score.

Putting two and two together, you can see how focusing on what we *can't* do (versus what we *can* do) conspires with conditions such as advertising, poverty, and lack of access to green space and healthy food to foster the poor health behaviors that prematurely age us. I've heard these "I can't" messages from countless people in the clinic, in the hospital, and even from patients I run into on the street. With little more than a shrug, so many people tolerate the erroneous beliefs that feed these behaviors for decades, allowing them to hijack what otherwise could have been a longer, more fruitful, and enjoyable life.

When we examine our "I can't" beliefs in a matter-of-fact, practical way, we start to realize that some of them are a little off, while others are flat-out wrong. It is particularly interesting to me that pessimism, which lends strength to our negative beliefs, is so often touted as being synonymous with realism, when in fact it may hold us back from seeing a realistic solution and actively moving toward that better reality. One of my professors in medical school, Dr. Alex Lickerman, author of *The Undefeated Mind: On the Science of Constructing an Indestructible Self,* used to tell me, "A candle can light up a cave that's been dark for a thousand years." The take-home: Regardless of how dark our own health situation has been and regardless of for how long, even the spark of one idea to do things differently can light our path to better health. So as we think about our own past experience — "I did x, y, and z for so long, the damage is already done" — we must be open to the possibility of new experience: "People change every day, and I can get help to change, too." Even if we failed before, things change, and we must try again and acknowledge every forward step.

STEP 5: FOLLOW TYPICAL DOCTOR ADVICE

We've all heard our doctor recite the litany of "no-brainer" steps to healthy aging, such as getting enough sleep, exercising regularly, eating a healthy diet, and, when appropriate, taking medication to control blood sugar, blood pressure, and blood cholesterol. While you may understand how im-

199

portant these steps are for heart health, it may surprise you to learn just how spot-on this advice is for healthy aging across all organ systems. Adhering to these basic tenets of preventive medicine also serve as important outlook guideposts. Exercise and sleep, in particular, support your outlook journey by stabilizing mood and boosting cognition, so I'll focus on these two aspects of typical doctor advice. A healthier attitude begets healthier action, which in turn begets a healthier attitude, propelling you in an "upward spiral" as Dr. Barbara Fredrickson, esteemed psychology researcher and author of *Positivity,* has aptly named this process.

Exercise

Evolutionarily speaking, movement and cognition go hand in hand: When we are moving, we are primed to think and to learn. Over millions of years, we had to learn quickly as we walked the earth, so movement jump-starts our brains as much as it gets our hearts pumping faster. Physical exercise encourages the birth of new neurons in the adult brain, termed *neurogenesis.* Research in mice also suggests that exercise further encourages these baby neurons to incorporate into existing networks, thus making them more functional and therefore useful for mental tasks.

How Exercise Can Reorient Our Outlook

If you need more motivation to get back on the treadmill — even if you're only standing on it at first — look no further than the mood-exercise link. You literally can walk, run, or bike your way to healthier outlook territory. Research on mice and men (and women) has demonstrated physical activity's clear benefits to our brain, both for helping us manage negative states of mind such as anxiety, sadness, and addiction cravings, and for improving our memory long term. One of the best compilations of the cognitive and emotional benefits of exercise is the 2008 book *Spark,* written by Harvard psychiatrist John Ratey, M.D. He describes how even those of us who are not clinically depressed can still benefit from the outlook-enhancing effects of regular physical activity. By "outlook-enhancing" I am referring to the way in which vigorous exercise seems to hit the reset button on our pessimistic and ruminative patterns of thinking that otherwise could result in unchecked anger, sadness, and frustration. For some, exercise may lead to adopting a more optimistic outlook. For others, exercise may confer the confidence to persist — in exercising and perhaps in other healthy behaviors. Persistence is a component of conscientiousness, which, like dispositional optimism, has been shown to predict better health and longevity.

While the scientific explanations for the beneficial outlook reorienting effects of physical activity have not been thoroughly worked out, existing evidence supports several mechanisms. First, a good old-fashioned sweat session probably increases neurotransmitters and other feel-good chemicals in specific areas of the brain that help us regulate our negative emotions. A recent study on stress in mice showed that unrestricted exercise on the Habitrail buffered the mice's ability to handle stress — and appeared to do so by ramping up the neuronal activity in two areas of their limbic system: the medial prefrontal cortex and the amygdala. Together, these two areas make up what neuroscientists term a *corticolimbic circuit,* which is thought to be evolutionarily critical for managing strong negative emotions. To be clear, negative emotions are important to alert us to potentially dangerous or otherwise important situations, but after we've heeded the warning call, they need to dissipate. We humans have corticolimbic circuits as well, and interestingly, they have been found to be dysfunctional in conditions such as clinical depression. For people who do suffer from clinical depression, anxiety, and other disorders, including ADHD and addiction, Dr. Ratey argues — and many doctors across the nation, including me, agree — that exercise should be prescribed just like a medicine, usually in combination with standard therapies for these conditions.

Though I myself have not been diagnosed with depression or anxiety (yet), I sure do run the outlook gamut, spending many an hour in fatalistic territory, which, as you know, doesn't feel good and makes it harder to get stuff done. During these times, if I can force myself to get up out of my chair and onto the mini-trampoline in my office to jump for fifteen or twenty minutes, I can feel this "medicine" working. Exercise literally blunts my rough emotional edges, shifting the content of my inner conversation toward less negative territory, allowing me to continue on with more peace, enthusiasm, and productivity than I had a few minutes before.

Exercise is a mood booster whether you are mentally healthy, suffering from a mood disorder, or somewhere in between. I tell myself and my patients to use exercise "on cue" whenever unhealthy outlook territory is close by. We discussed the borders of this territory in chapter 4, when I introduced Dr. Zindel Segal's concept of the "territory of depression" and my own adaptation, the "territory of relapse." Recall that both of these dangerous territories have chitchat patterns that we can recognize if we are paying attention to our inner conversation. The territory of relapse is, in part, characterized by thoughts of denial and apathy and may look and sound something like, "Oh, I don't really care about laying off the sauce — after all, I *like* drinking, and one cocktail isn't going to hurt me," along with that unmistakable tug of strong craving. This slippery slope is of course not limited to any one behavior, and you could just as easily imagine your own mental conversation around a quart of Häagen-Dazs or a cigarette in your hands.

Physical activity can temporarily catapult you out of the territories of depression, relapse, and other unsavory outlook addresses long enough to get your bearings and steer yourself in a different direction. And while any kind of movement is great, you'll get the most benefit from moderate and vigorous exercise. How can you gauge moderate or vigorous according to your fitness level? There are several rules of thumb that you've probably heard or even used. (As with any exercise program, it's important to check in with your doctor before starting, though I usually do not ask patients to make an appointment with me before they begin slow walking — that would be overkill.) During moderate activity (such as fast walking or easy jogging), your breathing rate and heart rate rise, and you may start to sweat. You are able to carry on a conversation but may not be able to belt out your favorite tunes. Your heart rate is generally in the zone of 60 to 70 percent of maximum heart rate. To calculate your maximum heart rate, subtract your age from 220. And for easy readings, you can purchase a heart-rate monitor for about fifty dollars from any sporting goods store. Vigorous activity means you're really hoofin' it to a level at which you are sweating and may not be able to carry on a full conversation. It gets your heart rate up to the range of 70 to 80 percent maximum. Again, these are ranges, and everyone's body, like everyone's outlook, is a little different. My purpose here is not to write a how-to on fitness. Rather, it is to entice you to begin — or continue — to move!

To get the immediate benefits of exercise, use it at will, just like you would call a trusted friend or counselor when you're in danger of reverting to unstable outlook territory. But don't assume you can run around the block once and be protected long term. Just like with medication, you have to "dose" yourself regularly, and ideally on the majority of days per week. Beyond the relatively quick relief from suffering that aerobic activity can provide, exercising regularly over time is like laying down emotional insulation. For all the reasons I've mentioned, including beneficial changes in brain chemistry and function, we are simply better able to handle outlook ups and downs when we are active. It's important to note that you do not have to have a life of luxury to reach this outlook guidepost. Except on rare occasions, I don't have a spare hour and a half to work out, shower, and change, so I do what I can with the time that I have, which is sometimes only fifteen minutes — a duration that I constantly strive to increase.

Exercise and Memory: Preventing Shrinkage

Exercise also protects the human hippocampus, a curved ridge deep in our forebrains that allows us to form, store, and process memory. In a 2011 study led by Dr. Kirk Erickson (formerly of the University of Illinois and now at the University of Pittsburgh), men and women ages fifty-five to eighty were randomized — akin to the flip of a coin — to two types of moderate-intensity exercise three days per week. One group was assigned to walking for forty minutes per day to reach the standard recommended target of 60 to 75 percent of maximal heart rate, and the other group was asked to perform a variety of stretching exercises. A trained exercise coach led the classes for both groups. The research participants underwent three types of testing before and after the year of exercise: structural MRI brain scans to measure the volume of several regions, including the hippocampus; cognitive testing, which included a spatial memory task in which the participants viewed dots on a screen and had to remember their location several seconds later; and measurement of serum brain-derived neurotrophic factor (BDNF), the biochemical equivalent of a "Scooby snack" for neurons that facilitates their birth, development, and integration into neural networks.

After a year, the data showed several

astounding results. First, the men and women who walked had larger hippocampi compared to when they started the study, while the hippocampi of those who only stretched actually *shrank.* By the way, here's a fun fact you may or may not want to know: In older adulthood, our hippocampi normally shrink about one percent every year, and this hippocampal shrinkage is in turn responsible for some of our cognitive decline as we age. But now we know we can do something as simple as regular walking to intervene on our own behalf.

Another exciting finding: Among the walkers, increases in blood levels of BDNF were correlated with increases in hippocampal volume. BDNF is particularly "tasty" to neurons in an area of the hippocampus called the dentate gyrus. What's more, these hippocampal volume and BDNF changes were directly related to the walkers' improved memory function. The bottom line? It was as if the walkers' hippocampi had *reverse-aged* by about two years, while the stretchers' hippocampi continued to diminish. And mind you, these research subjects were not young whippersnappers whose brains remained flexible through youth alone — they were the same age as or older than Victor (from chapter 1) and Helen (from chapter 2), providing clear evidence that you can influence how fast your memory ages — *even as an older person.* So how does this information change your perspective on exercise? I don't know about you, but it makes me want to put on my walking shoes and get going!

Sleep and Outlook

Something as basic as sleeping enough each night can also help you physiologically and psychologically stay *up.* The converse is also true, as we all know from experience: A lack of sleep for a period of time can cause our thoughts and feelings to spiral downward. Sleep deprivation in particular can send us into scary outlook territory. Even moderate sleep deprivation wreaks havoc with wide-ranging neuronal networks that allow us to perceive, think, and feel. What's more, you cannot restore all systems to normal simply by drinking coffee or taking other stimulants — even if a double shot of espresso opens your eyes a bit wider, some of those neurons remain sleepy until they can go nighty-night. So it is no surprise that when we are sleep deprived, we neither think nor emote as well as when we are rested, and our actions reflect the true state of our nervous system.

Some of my own toughest downward spirals have come during times when severe and prolonged sleep deprivation robbed me of my usually decent coping skills. For example, during my first year in medical school, my grandmother suffered a massive stroke, and I helped my mom care for her on the weekends. Totally new to medicine and the first in my family to enter the field, I was already worried enough about the scholastic work. When I then had to heap on the caretaking weekend shifts, it put me over the edge. These shifts began with a forty-five-minute drive south on the Dan Ryan Expressway, a notoriously dangerous strip of highway leading toward the old Chicago steel mills. This was an area where most of the men in my family had lived and worked since the early 1900s, so it had always had the historical appeal of going back in time to some of my roots. But instead of comfort on crossing the threshold of my grandma's row house, there was only agony as I watched this once-vibrant woman, who had relished weekly polka dancing for fifty years, spend half an hour fighting her way across her tiny kitchen and out onto the porch to light up and "pound her coffin pegs." Her keen insight into her strong addiction made it that much more frustrating to watch. While I loved my mother and grandmother and wanted to help, these weekends contributed to a downward outlook spiral, and what I needed to do at the time was protect myself better by admitting that I was not capable of going to medical school during the week and caregiving on the weekends. Collectively, the three of us were so physically and mentally exhausted that we could not see our way clear to the obvious solution, which was to hire a full-time caregiver. (Granted, finding a good one is sometimes much easier said than done.)

Several years later, during residency training, my husband (then my fiancé) and I found ourselves arguing nightly, which was unusual for us. At one point we even considered whether we were meant to get married, illustrating how difficult circumstances such as severe sleep deprivation and lack of recreation can mislead even reasonable people toward distinctly unreasonable decisions. Thankfully it dawned on us that we hadn't had a day off together in three months, and that we needed to reevaluate under more favorable living conditions. This was in the mid- to late 1990s, before there were mandated limits on residents' work hours. The grind of thirty-six-hour call shifts every fourth night for the better part of three years coupled with zero time spent together, had taken its toll on our perspective toward our upcoming marriage; we had both temporarily lost hope about our future together. But we didn't need to break up — we just needed some REM sleep, along with a chance to have lunch and watch a movie, go shopping, or take a walk together. There was nothing we could do in the short term to fix our long work hours, but we were able to appeal to our chief residents, who were in charge of making the schedules, to synchronize our days off wherever possible. That way we got to sleep in and schedule some fun activities, which instantaneously steered us toward a healthier perspective. If I had let the oppressive fatigue and isolation decimate my marriage plans, my life would be very different than it is today. Sometimes a combination of stabilizer steps is needed to get us back on track.

There are other consequences of not catching enough shut-eye that are equally detrimental, but that you cannot necessarily feel. Did you know that your pancreas needs a good night's sleep, too? When your pancreas is deprived of z's, its normally near-perfect hormonal calibration deteriorates, resulting in impaired glucose tolerance (higher blood sugar after meals), which can lead to weight gain, among other things. In one recent study of sleep restriction in which healthy people slept for just over four hours a night over a period of six days, the average blood sugar after a meal was 15 mg/dL higher than when they were sleeping longer. Their bodies were not able to clear the blood sugar as quickly, and their pancreases secreted one-third less insulin than they had at the beginning of the study, when they were rested. In less than one week of sleep deprivation, these young, healthy volunteers took on the metabolic profile of older people with prediabetes. As if that were not bad enough, their metabolism dropped by an average of 8 percent, which would be enough to result in a ten-pound weight gain over one year if the sleep deprivation continued. And that's not even taking into account how sleep deprivation stokes our appetite by increasing the hunger hormone, ghrelin, and lowering the fullness hormone, leptin.

STEP 6: REACH OUT FOR THE BENEFITS OF SOCIAL SUPPORT

If left completely to our own devices, sometimes we'll stumble, and need a friend, coach, guide, or some other steady force to reorient us. The help or support we get from other people in our network is termed *social support,* and it comes in many shapes and sizes, such as tangible support (someone to take you to the doctor), affectionate support (someone to hug you and tell you you're great), positive social interactions (someone with whom you can have a beer or see a show), emotional/informational support (someone to confide in), etc. Our family and friends can help insulate us from the myriad stressors in our lives.

We intuitively know this to be true, but scientists have also found proof of social network benefits in the laboratory. I have always been fascinated with how easy it is to experimentally ruffle someone's feathers (including my own) by putting them through a short public speaking or math test. Even though the research participants know it is all just an experiment, many of them still have a full-fledged fight-or-flight response. Specifically, the heart and blood pressure effects of stress are referred to as *cardiovascular reactivity.* This term encompasses high initial amplitude (blood pressure and heart rate skyrocket), prolonged recovery (blood pressure and heart rate take a long time to normalize), or both. Higher cardiovascular reactivity to stress has been linked to early atherosclerosis. What's even more interesting — and wonderful — is how the simple presence of a friendly person in the room can lessen this stress response.

I was on the receiving end of cardiovascular reactivity research one day during a graduate school class in psychophysiology. *Psychophysiology* is the scientific name for the study of how our psychology — what we think and feel — affects our physiology, which is essentially the subject of this entire book. I remember wearing a heart monitor and watching my own heart rate rise precipitously while I performed a mental stress task in front of the class. The task is called a Stroop, which involves naming the color of a word while ignoring the actual word; for example, answering "red" when the word *blue* is written in red ink. If you've never done a Stroop task, be warned: Even the easiest version is surprisingly harder than it sounds. I was classified as a "high stress responder," because the amount by which my heart rate and blood pressure rose in response to the experiment was above a certain threshold. And boy, could I feel it! Hot cheeks, pounding chest, sweaty palms, the whole bit. But remember that night on call when I was responsible for resuscitating two patients at the same time? When I put the pulse oximeter on my own finger, it showed my heart rate to be the speed of someone who might have been peacefully asleep on a warm beach. So what distinguished those two situations? First, that night in the hospital, I had supreme confidence. Having run countless codes before, I knew I could help those people, and was thrilled to do so. Second, I was among friends — my two fearless interns and a nurse whom I knew and trusted. In that instance, I was inhabiting some pretty sweet outlook digs.

The stress-buffering effects of friends do more than keep our heart rates low — they help us live more joyful, healthy lives. In some cases, social support may literally save our lives — for example, people diagnosed with breast cancer who have more social support have a lower risk of death, likely due to a combination of direct emotional benefits and the practical aspects of having someone to drive them to get their chemo and other therapies. The size of our social network does matter, in that being completely socially isolated is hazardous to your health. But having more family members and friends does not *always* translate into better health, especially when one considers that our social networks can also stress us out — a phenomenon the experts call *social strain.* What's so important is the strength of the bonds, and how much you perceive that your people lift you up.

A few really good friends are enough to buoy you in times of trouble. If you want more, there are of course lots of ways to make them — taking up a new hobby, joining a class or a book club, volunteering, or working in a community garden, to name a few. Online is an option, too, with proven beneficial health effects especially for behaviors such as eating a healthier diet and quitting smoking. If you already have "friends" but feel that they don't truly have your back, or that they seem to show up only out of obligation rather than out of any deeper bond, find new ones. Obviously, this is easier said than done for some of us introverts, but it's important to take even small steps to stay connected with people who truly nourish us. Our friends stop by to say hi, continue to keep up contact over time, and when it's needed, urge us to seek additional help.

Not surprisingly, aspects of our outlook are intimately tied to our relationships with other people. Optimism tends to foster strong and lasting bonds, while high cynical hostility — that tendency toward a deep-seated mistrust of others — undermines the stress-buffering effects of friendship. In one experiment, hostile people's cardiovascular reactivity did not diminish even in the presence of a friendly research staffer, suggesting that such an outlook interferes with gaining social benefits.

On the upside, a change in outlook can heavily influence our social support situation, which I know from firsthand experience. As a bookworm for the first two decades of life and an only child, I remember being in a state of social shock when I hit the clinical floors during my third year of medical school, when I was suddenly meeting tens of new patients and their family members daily, and interacting with myriad doctors, nurses, pharmacists, respiratory therapists, social workers, physical, occupational, and speech therapists, and other hospital staff. I had never talked to that many strangers each and every day for hours on end, taking only short breaks to eat, sleep, and use the bathroom.

While this high level of interaction at first seemed foreign, I saw that it was absolutely necessary in order to deliver optimal and integrated medical treatment, so I had no choice but to come out of my shell. There was something else I began to notice: Not only did I glean valuable medical information from chatting them up — I actually enjoyed connecting with them. Sometimes these connections have unexpectedly reached out and tapped me on the shoulder years later, as in the case of Ryan, a terminally ill cancer patient in his twenties, whom I cared for during my very first month of internship in the late 1990s. When I moved to Pittsburgh about eight years ago, all my books remained packed in boxes for months. One day as I was shelving them I flipped open the first volume of *The Norton Anthology of American Literature,* and out from between its tissue-paper-thin pages dropped a hauntingly beautiful note I had not seen in years, written in blue ink on the back of a piece of paper torn from Ryan's hospital menu and stamped with the room number, date, and his name. "Thanks for everything, Dr. Tindle," it read. "I'll look all you guys up when I come back. — Ryan."

At the time, Ryan, who had undergone a failed course of chemotherapy for leukemia, had been hospitalized because of low blood counts. A favorite patient among our house staff, he was witty, friendly, and good-looking, and on the outside his body looked healthy despite the battle raging inside; his bald head, which could easily pass for a bold

219

military look, was the only tip. On the eve of the weekend when Ryan was meant to be released, we were heartbroken to see the temperature on his chart. He had a neutropenic fever (a fever in the setting of a drastically suppressed immune system), which could have been due to tumor, serious infection, both, or something else. He couldn't safely leave the hospital. My resident reached out and put his hand on Ryan's shoulder. "Sorry, man, we have to keep you." After everything he had been through, Ryan told us he completely understood. But it was still hard for me to think about him sitting in that room alone for the duration of the weekend, longing to be outside.

After rounds I ran back to the call room and grabbed the anthology, which I'd stashed there in hopes that I would be able to read a few lines now and then, and handed it to him. Long before the advent of the iPad, a good book was a welcome oasis from deserted late-night hospital hallways stretching clear out to the horizon. This was my way (an introvert's way) of connecting with a patient, and to this day I see how meaningful such outreach can be. He must have read that anthology cover to cover before the day he was finally able to walk outside and catch the last bits of summer.

Ryan passed away the following year. When I saw his note it was as if I was again a twenty-six-year-old intern, standing at Ryan's bedside and witnessing the strength of one beautiful person's spirit.

Being carried back to earlier experiences of patients like Ryan — people whom I considered friends and who, by virtue of my being their doctor, allowed me to witness the sometimes inspiring, sometimes terrifying details of their lives — helps keep me in positive outlook territory. Here was a man facing illness and death with such buoyancy, grace, and manners — a thank-you note! — that I cannot help but be encouraged to face my own adversities, which are currently not so dire, with a similar tenor. Reaching out to these people has helped shape who I am today — I am more aware of suffering, more grateful for health wherever I see it, and more committed to doing whatever possible to promote it widely. I would not have been able to look inside their lives without edging out of my comfort zone to engage and explore, and through my relationships with these patients and their families, I realized I was often gaining as much as I gave. So while introverts provide an invaluable perspective on the world (*Quiet* author Susan Cain is right), for those of us turtles, there are benefits to creating an "extro" version of ourselves. Fortunately, our outlook is more fluid than we think — a concept we'll discuss more in the next chapter — and there may be times when it is especially malleable, rendering us more open to change.

You may also find that the outlook of your friends can start to wear off on you. Aspects of outlook do appear to be somewhat contagious. Drs. Nicholas Christakis and James Fowler, authors of *Connected: How Your Friends' Friends' Friends Affect Everything You Feel, Think, and Do,* have shown that our states of mind (such as happiness) and health conditions (such as obesity and smoking) pass through social networks like propagating waves. Certain individuals who are at the center of a network can have more influence over a greater number of people than those who are more socially isolated. It's important to understand that this wave moves slowly — over decades rather than weeks or months — so it is not like your friends and family can change you overnight (or you them). Nevertheless, you may have noticed your own inner conversation start to temporarily darken when you spend a lot of time with friends who are particularly pessimistic, cynical, or neurotic. On the other hand, being around people who are more *up* often has the opposite effect. I can think of several instances in which I purposely tried to avoid or embrace certain people based on their outlook tendencies.

How Language Helps Us Connect with Each Other

It may seem obvious, but it bears mentioning. Words, whether they are written, spoken, or sung, can transport us across time and space to reunite with people, places, and things we love and subsequently boost our mood and help us feel connected and comforted. It is through poetry that I most often remember my father, a teacher and poet, who died at the tender age of fifty-two from metastatic pancreatic cancer. Sitting in a chair next to the fireplace in his home in central California, he used to recite lines from a Robinson Jeffers poem, "The Bloody Sire," which he had come across during his studies at the venerable Iowa Writers' Workshop, where my parents met: *What but the wolf's tooth whittled so fine/The fleet limbs of the antelope?/What but fear winged the birds, and hunger/Jewelled with such eyes the great goshawk's head?* "You must promise you will remember this," he told me, "for its sheer beauty." Minutes before he passed away, my father recited from memory W. H. Auden's "In Praise of Limestone." Now I regularly read Jeffers, W. H. Auden, and other poets my parents knew and admired, to rekindle his memory.

We can also use language and customs to reconnect with roots of our entire culture. The Oglala Lakota on the Pine Ridge Reservation in southern South Dakota and other members of the Sioux nation have done just that to counter powerful forces that have devastated their physical, mental, and cultural health. People living on the Pine Ridge Reservation now suffer rates of poverty, infant mortality, suicide, and alcoholism that are three to six times the U.S. national average, not to mention extraordinary rates of obesity and diabetes. Their average life expectancy (66.6 years) is also ten years shorter than the U.S. national average (76.5). Only in a few other places in the U.S. (such as the inner city) can you find numbers that approach this level of social decimation. Rates of liver disease among Pine Ridge Sioux, fueled by alcoholism and obesity, are more than twelve times the U.S. national average. It is not shocking that they have continued to fight the sale of millions of cans of beer annually right outside the reservation borders.

Facing such overwhelming conditions and the widespread fatalism they engender, how do the Pine Ridge Sioux cope? As resident activist Alex White Plume stated during an August 2012 interview with journalist Alexandra Fuller for *National Geographic,* "Do you know what saved me from becoming a cold-blooded murderer? My language saved me. There is no way for me to be hateful in my language. It's such a beautiful, gentle language. It's so peaceful." To revisit the metaphor of the two wolves from chapter 3, speaking his native language was one way Alex White Plume was able to "feed the wolf" that best benefited him and his community. Slowly, the Sioux are rebuilding their community through their traditional stories, dances, and ceremonies — all centered around their own language and the more universal language of their sacred land. Whatever our heritage, we can home in on traditions of our family and our culture that bring us together and remind us of our purpose. As I demonstrated with my poetry example, even the smallest act of connection can be powerful. In the following section, you'll see how profoundly a connection with land and other aspects of the natural world sustain our outlook.

STEP 7: GET A HEALTHY DOSE OF GREEN: CULTIVATE YOUR MICROENVIRONMENT

Research shows that your physical environment can affect your outlook — and your health — in positive ways. Spending time in open green space, for example, has been linked to better health, from greater psychological well-being to lower blood pressure and even longer life. Researchers are still sussing out exactly how nature nurtures our body and mind, but certainly the fact that we typically move more when outside is part of the equation. Being in a natural setting also tends to calm and quiet the mind. I'm using the term *microenvironment* to underscore that while you may not be able to change the entire environment, you do have a say in where and when you spend some of your time, a fact you can use toward the goal of healthy aging.

Your microenvironment is not only the physical environs that surround you at home, at work, during recreation, and everywhere in between but also your psychosocial milieu — made up of the people you hang out with and the neighborhood(s) you frequent. I think of the microenvironment as the intersection of our social network and our surroundings, both built and natural. In *Urban Place: Reconnecting with the Natural World,* editor and anthropologist Peggy Bartlett convincingly demonstrates how even small outposts of the plant kingdom such as your favorite tree, neighborhood park, or national park or forest enhance your experience, whether you live in an urban, suburban, or rural setting. Not only does contact with the natural world support our physical and mental health, she shows us, but it also fosters stronger social bonds and builds community, in part by getting us outside to move and interact with others. By the way, our community includes our animals, too, many of whom love to be outside feeling the wind on their fur, feathers, or scales.

Whether you are tilling soil in a community garden in Detroit or biking through Central Park in Manhattan, feeling sand and water wash over your feet as you stare out over the Pacific Ocean or sitting at your kitchen table feeling the smooth, waxy contours of a jade plant, you are "dosing" yourself with Mother Nature's medicine. In fact, the salutary effects of green spaces, including open tracts of green land such as fields and parks, are so powerful that they actually buffer some of the devastating health consequences of poverty, one of the most well-established risk factors for poor health and early death.

In a 2008 landmark article published in *The Lancet,* Drs. Richard Mitchell and Frank Popham studied the population of England and found that people who had the most access to green spaces had the smallest differences between rich and poor in the risk of death overall, whereas among people who had the least access to green spaces, the gap between rich and poor in the risk of death was much greater. The results also held true for death specifically due to cardiovascular disease, a leading cause of death in developed nations and a condition that is known to be influenced by both physical activity and stress. Importantly, the researchers found that access to green space did not matter for other causes of death such as lung cancer (primarily caused by cigarettes) or suicide (primarily caused by severe depression), which were not expected to be affected by such access. Taken together, these results provide compelling evidence that when it comes to some of the most common causes of illness and death, getting to green is good for your health.

So you can see why I am recommending that you infuse your microenvironment with as much green as possible. Clearly, not everyone has unfettered access. But to the extent that you can, try to get to natural spaces, whether they are across the street or two or three neighborhoods over. If you are able, try to weave your green time throughout the week rather than compressing it into a weekend day or infrequent vacation. Throughout my own workweek, I do what I can on lunch breaks, often taking a walk to the gardens of the nearby Phipps Conservatory. On days when leaving for lunch is not possible, I at least look out my window — luckily now I have a view, which wasn't always the case — and admire the greenery surrounding the conservatory while making a mental note to try to get there the next day.

On weekends, my husband and I take the kids and the dogs for longer walks in downtown Pittsburgh, where the Allegheny and the Monongahela merge to form the Ohio River, or through Hartwood Acres and North Park, two beautiful green spaces farther outside the city. These walks give our family the opportunity to exercise and enjoy nature at the same time.

Muscovites understand the microenvironment concept as well as any of us, as journalist Cathy Newman described in her 2012

National Geographic piece on the Russian dacha, or summer cottage. One-third of all Russians own a dacha, and for many of them, the one-tenth of an acre plot of land offers more than a weekend escape from city life — it is a portal to reconnect with the earth, cultivating nothing less than spiritual survival along with the vegetables that have for centuries sustained millions of Russians during severe food shortages. As one dacha owner put it, "At the end of the day I'm tired and stressed. Then I come to the dacha and put my hands in the soil and touch the earth — I touch the soil and bad things go away."

Regardless of our heritage, it is easy to feel inspired in nature. A few years ago I read a moving article in the *Chicago Tribune* that told the story of an agnostic advertising sales executive named John Lionberger, who had journeyed north to the frozen Boundary Waters of Minnesota on an Outward Bound–sponsored dogsledding trip. Standing in subzero temperatures, he found himself inexplicably "bathed in warmth," a phenomenon he came to recognize as a soothing, even spiritual presence. One day several months later, while he was sitting in the library, hemming and hawing about what it all meant and what he should do next, he again perceived the same presence. He was inspired to found Renewal in the Wilderness, an outfit that organizes outdoor trips designed to help people develop their spirituality through contact with nature.

We can be inspired by the natural world even if we don't "know exactly what a prayer is," says the poet Mary Oliver in "The Summer Day." In fact, she argues, establishing a connection with nature is key to fully living our "one wild and precious life." This connection to the natural world comes in many forms. For me, it came through study of the human body, taking shape one day during college while I was sitting in Mammalian Biology class listening to an in-depth lecture on embryology. I already knew that each developing human goes through some, though not all, of the major evolutionary stages preceding it. For example, both chick and human embryos develop and then discard the gill slits of their common ancestor. But when my professors — a dynamic husband and wife duo — taught us the specifics of how our very organs reflect this evolutionary history, I was forever hooked. The kidneys that work tirelessly to clean our blood, regulate blood pH and pressure, and stimulate red blood cell growth are actually preceded by more rudimentary kidneys reminiscent of our biological history — the pronephros, the mesonephros, and the metanephros, which are successively created and mostly broken down to make room for what later become the kidneys we are born with. I remember being in awe and thinking, "So much has gone into these kidneys! They need to be preserved and protected!" Before that day, although I had intellectually understood the process, I had never considered how valuable it rendered each and every organ and body: Each one of us is a repository for much of the collective biology of the planet. To me, this is precious and, in the words of my patient Helen, "worth taking care of." Whatever spurs us on, we must reach an attitude latitude that allows us to live this truth, both for ourselves and for those we love.

6
HOW OTHERS TRAVEL: CASE HISTORIES OF THE OUTLOOK GUIDES

You may be wondering: Is our outlook a product of nature or nurture? Research shows us that it's both, and that up to fifty percent is genetic. This means that we do get some of our outlook, along with eye and hair color, from our parents. In addition, more recent science has begun to fine-tune which genes may be associated with which traits. A study at UCLA found that a gene encoding the receptor for the hormone oxytocin is related to traits such as optimism. Oxytocin has myriad effects on our social functioning but is best known for its role in parent-child bonding, and has been simplistically dubbed the "love hormone." Carriers of the A allele, a genetic variant of this oxytocin receptor gene, had lower levels of optimism relative to those with two copies of the G allele, another variant. For those of us whose genes don't foster traits favoring healthy aging, it may seem like we're already starting with one hand tied behind our back. But when we look at it from the optimistic standpoint, that's actually not the case. If our genes determine less than half of our outlook, then we have control over more than half. So the question is, what forces can guide us *up*?

We arrive as babies at a distinct set of outlook coordinates that have been determined primarily by our DNA, because the only experience we've had up to that point is our brief time in the womb environment. As we grow, our outlook is strongly shaped by our experiences — the fabric of our daily lives, woven in part by our interpersonal relationships and our socioeconomic status — from childhood through early adulthood. Until recently, personality had long been thought to fully gel somewhere between age twenty and thirty, remaining steadfast thereafter. But now those theories are beginning to soften as scientists find that traits can continue to change to a certain extent once we reach adulthood. If you took a bunch of psychological questionnaires to characterize your Point A at age forty and then took them again at age fifty, you would see that Point A had changed, kind of like looking at two photographs of yourself snapped ten years apart. These changes in our outlook are not unlike the normal flux of other bodily systems, and may be just as imperceptible to us. In our day-to-day lives even portions of our bodies that we regard as steadfast, including our very backbone, are changing minute by minute. Through the work of osteoclasts (cells that break down bone), osteoblasts (cells that build up bone), and osteocytes (cells that maintain bone matrix), our entire skeleton turns over about every decade.

When it comes to outlook change, we adjust rather than replace, and just how much a person's outlook changes over the course of her life is a point of hot debate among experts in the field. Pioneering psychologists Robert McCrae and Paul Costa, who founded the Big Five model of personality, originally conceptualized personality as a relatively stable trait after young adulthood, and have produced evidence to support this view. On the other hand, there is evidence that even in adulthood, our personalities continue to grow and change with us. Dr. Carol Dweck, an established psychology researcher at Stanford and author of *Mindset: The New Psychology of Success* has thoughtfully and convincingly synthesized existing research to explain the flexible nature of our personalities and their capacity for change. Addressing the 2007 Annual Convention of the Association for Psychological Science, she emphasized how "[b]eliefs matter, beliefs can be changed, and when they are, so too is personality."

Everyone agrees that personality traits naturally change during the first three decades of life, but information about changes over longer periods remains less understood. Recently, Dr. Sarah Hampson, personality psychologist and senior scientist at the Oregon Research Institute, and her team studied conscientiousness and other personality traits in ten-year-old kids (as assessed by their school-teachers) who now, forty years later, have turned the big five-oh. (I briefly introduced this study in chapter 1.) Only a very small percentage of the conscientiousness levels of the ten-year-olds remained stable into middle age, underscoring big changes over those four decades. Even after allowing for methodologic issues such as having only two measurements in forty years and comparing teachers' ratings at one time point with participants' self-ratings at another (common in research that spans the life course), we can see that change happens. Thus, rather than permanently hardening like clay or rock, our character traits may be more fluid than we think. Further, Dr. Hampson notes that our traits are naturally more apt to change as we meet major life milestones, including going to college, getting married, having a baby, and even getting sick. Except for major illness, most of these things do tend to happen in our twenties and thirties — and for some of us late bloomers, forties and beyond — which may be one reason our outlook is more apt to change during these years. So the things we typically think of as life benchmarks are also outlook benchmarks: Having a baby, for example, goes thankfully hand in hand with greater conscientiousness.

As I've stressed already, outlook change, whether inadvertent or intentional, does not necessarily mean that one must become, or even *could* become, a totally different person — although it may seem at times that your adolescent has been invaded by the body snatchers. Rather, as we go through life we take on new characteristics and shed old ones, often without even trying, and without altering who we are essentially. What will be very interesting to study in the future is the extent to which conscientiousness and other promising character traits can be cultivated to maximize healthy aging.

Then there are the events that catalyze the process of outlook change, such as catastrophes and other frame-shifting events, whether they are good or bad. But there is no rule that says you must be crushed by life in order to learn from it, and if at all possible, it's a much easier path to move to safer ground on your outlook globe *before* major physical and/or psychological upheaval. This is not to say that proactive attitudinal change offers immunity to the emotional fallout from accidents, job loss, and other major setbacks. But considering that optimism, conscientiousness, agreeableness, and other "healthy" character traits help us field life's curveballs, my view is: Embrace them now. Admittedly, I've been influenced by my experiences, including the heart surgery, which set much of my outlook trek in motion.

There are people all around us who can help show us the way. I refer to them as the "outlook guides" because they act as a compass, showing us what to do and how to do it. Their advice complements and underscore the guideposts we've already visited. This chapter includes three guides who have influenced me, and who continue to support many others to move *up*. (I could not fit all of my guides into one book.) They show us that while the proverbial apple may not fall far from its tree, between our own efforts and their guidance, it can roll a long way.

WISHWA KAPOOR, M.D.: ONE MAN'S QUEST TO "BROADEN AND BUILD"

I found out just how far the apple can roll under the most surprising of circumstances: a meeting with my boss. To me, he has always been the somewhat severe but benevolent leader, Dr. Wishwa Kapoor, chief of the Division of General Internal Medicine at the University of Pittsburgh and vice chairman of the Department of Medicine, along with numerous other titles reflecting his complete integration into the university and the medical center over the past twenty-five years. Sitting in his office one day during my annual review session (not exactly the most relaxing of situations), he made a comment that tipped me off to his status as an extraordinary attitudinal globetrotter. "I am very optimistic, but I didn't start out that way," he told me as we reviewed the results of my study showing that optimists have fewer heart attacks and live longer than pessimists. Having only seen his confident and upbeat attitudinal Point B — which so often seemed miles above my own mercurial outlook — I *had* to know more about his Point A and the journey *up*. I finally persuaded him to tell the remarkable story of how he traversed two globes: first planet Earth and then planet Outlook. He initially left his home in Afghanistan, and over time and circumstances broadened his perspective, remodeled his somewhat gloomy childhood outlook, and built a brilliant life. He is a living example of what happens when a person, as Dr. Barbara Fredrickson terms it, "broadens and builds."

"I grew up in the Hindu ghetto in Kabul," he began. "It was basically a small community of Hindus — mud houses, open sewers, no running water, no toilets, a pretty primitive situation. And I was one of six kids in my immediate family." They lived in a small house, along with his uncle and five cousins, and "when my brother got married, he brought his bride to the same house." There were many aspects of his childhood that Dr. Kapoor loved, most notably the continual presence of family, being integrated into the neighborhood, and other children to talk, laugh, and play with: "The community was very close-knit, and so you grew up to be part of the community, to do things the way everything was done. It was very traditional." Dr. Kapoor never minded certain traditions, such as dressing and eating *exactly* like everyone else, but there were other facets of the rigid environment that he found increasingly difficult to accept as he grew older.

For starters, the idea that you could improve your lot — or that you'd even question it at all — was virtually nonexistent in his community. He also was part of a culture of negativity featuring inertia toward personal change, either outward or inward. "People were pessimistic. They didn't see how they could improve themselves. When you grew up in that environment, a lot of people didn't think about the future; it just didn't occur to them. And if you don't think about [the future], you just float." He remembers how for years his self-image — along with hope of any kind of achievement — was shaped by a derision that seemed built into everyday conversation. He was often compared with his cousins and "always told that I was really not that good, didn't do well in school, didn't really do anything well." Nor was the psychological environment entirely safe outside his neighborhood, either in school or on the street, where he was "one Hindu among many

Muslims." While he had many Muslim friends, the underlying cultural differences sometimes made for strained interpersonal relationships and prejudice even during that time of relative peace in the 1950s and '60s.

It was a foregone conclusion that he would take over his father's small shop as an adult. Employment opportunities were severely limited, and people typically carried on what their parents had started, no questions asked. Dr. Kapoor remained what he describes as "a mediocre student" who was thoroughly disengaged from the learning process: sitting at the back of the room, memorizing what he was told, and suffering the occasional physical punishment if he didn't know something. "I sat there and did things, but it just didn't click." Even more oppressive than the academic ennui — and the bleak professional horizon it promised — was the lack of autonomy in choosing a spouse: "The thing that was really problematic was who you were supposed to marry. As a young child there was already somebody arranged for me."

There were clearly some very powerful forces — economic, social, and political — conspiring to keep the young Kapoor and his outlook down. But in his mind, he firmly knew he didn't want the life his parents and his entire society expected him to have. The fact that he even dared to think such thoughts underscores his feisty, questioning, almost rebellious disposition. Despite this growing defiance, his trajectory seemed to be heading inexorably toward fulfilling the very traditions he internally resisted. And then when he was thirteen, something *did* click. "It was about ninth grade when I suddenly became very, very interested in learning. And I can't tell what it was. I guess it was just maturation, growing up, and probably also seeing what the future was going to be like. If I didn't get educated, what would I do? I would be working with my father at his store buying and selling things." His mind raced, simultaneously desperate and proactive: "I need to get out of this! How can I get out of this?" He saw one possible future laid out before him and believed he could have something different. As he mulled over these questions, his remarkably strong sense of agency rose to the surface: "How can I *create* opportunities?" Gradually the answer came. "And what I was realizing was that I needed to work on education. Education was the clear ladder. There was no other ladder. And so I became pretty good in school — I did well that year."

He was poised to enter the next school year as the number three student out of a couple hundred kids, and that's when things really got interesting. The American Field Service, a worldwide exchange student program of which I am also a graduate, was offering the number one and two students in each class the chance to spend a year in the United States. As number three, Dr. Kapoor would not have been eligible to try out but for a twist of fate: The number one student in his level skipped ahead to the next grade, opening the door wide for Dr. Kapoor to step through. In this case, chance truly did favor the prepared mind: "The best thing that ever happened to me was that that guy moved up." So in 1965 this "shy, sheltered seventeen-year-old" boy, who had barely left the city limits of Kabul, now "boarded a plane to New York, took a bus to Detroit, got into a convertible driven by a beautiful forty-year-old woman — the mother of the family — and was taken to a beach."

Arriving on a warm August day in his new home of Allegan, Mich., population of about five thousand, where most people had never even heard of Afghanistan, the term *culture shock* could not begin to describe his reaction. Getting out of the car and laying eyes on the family's cabin by the lake, where everyone had gathered in their beach-wear, he felt as if he had been transported to another world. "It was the year that I really grew up," he remembers. "You know, a lot of people were very good to me. They contributed a lot. It was a year of significant maturation. It was a transformative year." Everything was new, from clothes to food to gender relations, not to mention immense pressure on this most introverted of intro-verts to become a veritable ambassador for his country. "I was a celebrity in town. . . . I had to stand up in front of the class and make presentations to the school. . . . I was on display." Looking back, this was a good experience for him, yet at the time, every public appearance sent him into panic mode. Compounding this crisis was the coed environment: "Women are sort of hid-den in Afghanistan, so you really don't have a real relationship except with your sisters, sisters-in-law, mother, and cousins." Over time he learned to relate to girls and women as friends, attended Friday night basketball games and dances, and even took a date to senior prom. And how did all that go? He can only laugh. "It was all very . . . *transfor-mative.*"

He also took on some pretty tough classes,

even though at that point he had only studied English to a grade school level — his fifth language after Punjabi at home and Farsi, Pashto, and Arabic at school. Luckily he not only had an outstanding English teacher at school but had a second professor at home. His host mother, Penny, was an accomplished Mark Twain scholar, and she helped him with his homework every weeknight for the entire year. After so many years of having been "a pretty nervous kid who just wanted to do well," he now began to feel the power of his own intellectual engines. He wasn't only building intellectual capital; he was also learning to see things through other people's eyes, a vantage point that, as you can imagine, was very different from the collectivist perspective of his earlier youth.

After a year, he returned home and finished the last few months of his senior year in Kabul, graduating as the valedictorian. He subsequently aced the university entrance exams and now had the choice of medicine or engineering: Things were definitely looking up. Over the course of just one year, he had gained a new perspective, brought on in part by new training and new experiences. As I alluded to in chapter 2, training — or educational resources — can go a long way toward reorienting our outlook, by bringing us knowledge and confidence, which in turn often help us see things differently. These rapid and profound changes were likely possible because he was so young and his outlook so malleable, underscoring how important it is to give kids opportunities to start building a healthy outlook as early as possible. For the first time, he dared to embrace the idea that he had a say in his own destiny.

But he had to face certain facts upon reentering Afghan society: "I was totally different. I didn't *fit* anymore. . . . I didn't think the same way, I didn't act the same way. I'm sure my parents were not happy that I had changed so much." Along with the several-degree shift in extroversion that he had undergone came a newfound and usually unwelcome ability to say what was on his mind. "The focus in the community was, 'How can you get settled in your life?' By that they meant marriage, kids, and a job — stable work. I really didn't want to do any of that stuff. I certainly didn't want to get married." In contrast to what was expected of him, he held another vision firmly in mind: "My focus totally was, 'How can I get back someplace where I can get a really good education?' " He waited for an opportunity to again study in the West, and soon saw his chance. One of his engineering professors at Kabul University recognized talent in the young Kapoor and offered to arrange a scholarship for him to finish his degree in the American Midwest.

With about six months remaining before he was scheduled to leave, he kept his plans from his family, for fear that they might be thwarted. "I had to navigate this very carefully," he said. If his parents knew of his plans, they would force him to get married before leaving. "They had absolute power. That's one of the amazing things — that when you are in that culture, the parents have absolute power. They can do *anything*. And in that culture, I *could not resist*. The only way I could resist — and renege on their promissory note of marriage — was if I was not physically there. And I could then write a letter, or I could say [from a safe distance], 'I'm not going to marry.' " And it was not only his parents, but the entire social structure that he would have to stand up to. "My parents, brothers, uncles, my cousins — *everybody* — so I had to navigate it very well. I told my parents two days before [leaving], and they were *really* upset." He remembers throwing down the gauntlet. " 'Here is my passport, here's the ticket —

I'm going!' " Despite his parents' shock and ire, there was no way they could mobilize a wedding in a day. "It caused a lot of turmoil, but I left and went to St. Louis."

With opportunity comes the burden of choice, and making this choice — to put his own needs as a human being over and above the wishes of his parents and community — must have felt like trying to escape the gravitational pull of a region that for him had become a black hole (albeit a beloved one). In deciding to leave, he wasn't choosing optimism per se, but instead was in hot pursuit of educational capital, which offered him not only greater confidence and a strong sense of self, but limitless possibilities. His optimism, which grew with each little bit of success, was actually an unintended consequence, although it's worth noting that he had enough positive expectation to even try in the first place. It was only later, when he saw how his attitude was changing, that he realized the power of this new outlook. "I had grown up with a sense of being a failure. As I succeeded in many things, my confidence increased and it improved my self-image. It led to a sense that it is possible to do whatever I wanted to if I devoted enough effort."

He excelled at Washington University, and

realized his parents' worst fear: He met and married a Western woman. Eventually, his parents accepted his choices. "They were good to me," he remembers. "They didn't disown me." Looking back on his journey from the vantage point of his current position, Dr. Kapoor recognizes that statistically speaking, he is what is called an outlier. This term, as applied to extraordinary people, has been made famous by Malcolm Gladwell in his book of the same name. Not only has he landed standard deviations beyond where the expected trajectory would have put him, but his unique path is a product of his own outlook and some extraordinary circumstances. "If you look at my life, and where I came from, I should not be doing this." But before you write off his experience as a one-in-a-million shot, consider what actually makes a set of circumstances extraordinary. Sometimes, it's simply the fact that we seize the opportunities as they come. As Dr. Kapoor illustrates, doing this takes foresight and enough confidence to lean forward and take that first step. It's not *only* our outlook and not *only* our circumstances that propel us forward or hold us back, but *both*.

Dr. Kapoor also notes how these attitudinal changes took years, and occurred at a

glacial pace that was at times barely percep-
tible to him. "I grew up pessimistic, and I
stayed pessimistic for a long time, and I
think my attitudes probably changed about
twenty to thirty years ago as I became more
comfortable." In other words, he really
began to notice that he was thinking about
things differently as some of the major life
milestones fell into place. He had purchased
a home, had two children of his own, and
had been on the medical faculty for several
years before he started to feel truly settled.
Not one who was normally given to self-
praise, he now had no choice but to recognize the impressive academic and social
capital he had built, and this conscious
acknowledgment of success further galva-
nized his belief in what he could accomplish.
But if he had to choose one attitudinal
inflection point that set the rest of the
course in motion: "I think the major growth
was probably that year in Michigan. I
changed a lot. You know, taking somebody
and putting them someplace else is like taking a raw egg and putting it in hot water —
you get a boiled egg!" But even now, as a
sixty-four-year-old "boiled egg," he recognizes that "there are [still] pessimistic
streaks."

This is to be expected for any outlook

traveler. Remember, the goal is not to wipe your slate clean — we are talking about personality *adjustment,* not transplant, to better our health and aging. Dr. Kapoor finds himself lapsing back into old patterns now and then. "You may not believe it, but I've continued to struggle. . . . I zigzag." Many of us can relate to zigzagging. We don't look with the exact same eyes on the same situation on any given day. Perhaps I caught a glimpse of Dr. Kapoor's outlook, somewhat similar to my own, even before I knew his whole story, and that's what drew me to him in the first place. Here's something else that may surprise you. Despite creating and following that pathway out of Kabul, traveling halfway around the world, securing a phenomenal education, marrying the woman he fell in love with and having a family, and enjoying a wildly successful career in medicine — in short, building an entire life for himself from scratch — from his perspective, much of his outlook hasn't changed. This should give hope to those of you who may still be skeptical of whether you can accomplish meaningful outlook travel. "You know, in many ways, a lot of things are not that different from when I was little, because the personalities don't change that much. The fundamentals don't change that much." And what are those fundamentals? "The reservedness, the introversion, spending time reflecting, thinking." He may be comfortable getting up and speaking in a room full of five hundred people now, but the introversion that drives him to sit quietly and channel his brain power to the benefit of so many people has remained intact.

While Dr. Kapoor himself may not feel that he has changed much, he has managed enough outlook travel to alter his own destiny. Not only was he the first of his entire Hindu community to "make it out" and achieve such success, but these geographical and attitudinal travels literally saved his life: "Where would I be? If I had stayed in that environment, I would be either dead — or if I were lucky, I would be driving a taxi in D.C. A lot of these [taxi drivers] are really smart; it's just that they didn't have opportunities to advance." Or maybe some didn't seize those opportunities, at least not for themselves. Dr. Kapoor highlights something fascinating about outlook that he learned talking to other immigrants: "If you take the time to talk to them, many of them are pessimists. And they are pessimists because they just have been through such horrific things, and they are here [in the U.S.], but they are really hoping that things will work out for their kids, not for themselves. Their own life is not great. They want to make sure their kids do well." Whatever hope they have burns for their children. This is a critical point. Up until now, I have characterized our outlook as a tool to enhance our *own* healthy aging, but it is more than that. The further we travel on our own outlook globe, the greater the consequences for those around us, starting with our family and the people closest to us.

Consider how Dr. Kapoor's outlook travels have altered the destiny of his children, grandchildren, extended family (now scattered across Europe, India, and Asia), and countless young physicians and scientists. And don't think he doesn't let his children know it! "I tell my kids, 'You guys should be very grateful!' " (They are.) So even as Dr. Kapoor zigzagged, he was still moving in a healthy direction, and little by little he has been able to let go of the fatalistic tendencies of his youth, learn to envision his future with hope instead of resignation, and embrace the opportunities that have spurred him on to a life of learning, teaching, and healing. And just because his case is a model illustration for how attitudinal change facilitates healthy aging, it does not mean these benefits are out of reach for the rest of us. On the contrary, his life bears testimony to the fact that we *can* change, and while doing so, still remain ourselves. Often, it helps to employ trained outlook guides to explicitly show the rest of us travelers where to go, step by step. The next two people we'll meet are on the front lines of attitudinal change — people who make their living helping others reach more fertile outlook ground.

CHRIS GERMER, PH.D.: THE MEDICINE OF SELF-COMPASSION

I first met Dr. Germer, a clinical psychologist specializing in mindfulness and compassion-based psychotherapy, when I took his class during my years of fellowship training. He is a founding member of the Institute for Meditation and Psychotherapy, a clinical instructor at Harvard Medical School, and coeditor of *Wisdom and Compassion in Psychotherapy: Deepening Mindfulness in Clinical Practice, Mindfulness and Psychotherapy,* and *The Mindful Path to Self-Compassion: Freeing Yourself from Destructive Thoughts and Emotions.* But to me and many others who know him, he is Chris, the outlook go-to guy, always at the ready to hear his clients' stories, sit and breathe with them, and deliver sage advice that is as effective as it is kind. Chris's efforts center on teaching people to cultivate self-compassion, which he defines as the intention to care for and generate goodwill toward oneself. If you're thinking that cultivating goodwill is relevant only around the holidays, think again: We are actually hardwired to feel content, connected, and safe at all times because it ensures our very survival.

Chris draws on the work of Dr. Paul Gilbert, veteran psychologist, researcher, and author of *The Compassionate Mind: A New Approach to Life's Challenges,* to explain how the parts of our brain that allow us to generate compassion may be the most critical of the three neural networks that promote our survival — fight-or-flight (running from a lion, for example), pleasure and reward (seeking out food, water, a mate), and affiliation with others. Most people are quite familiar with the first two, but the compassion-generating system, which has been associated with the release of the hormone oxytocin, is one we now, as a species, want to enhance: When it's most active, we feel safe and comfortable with ourselves and others. Through compassion for ourselves and others, this system brings us closer together, and has thus been termed our *affiliative* system, because it helps us attach to one another in healthy ways. The affiliative network is especially critical for mammals, whose survival depends on parent-infant bonding. When we are babies cooing to our parents, we want their affiliative system to be as strong as possible, because it ensures our continued development and survival. Later, when we are the parents cooing back at our baby, a strong affiliative system brings us greater contentment and from an evolutionary perspective, ensures the survival of the species. As we've already seen, these bonds with family and friends continue to support our mental and physical health at any age.

Chris points out another reason to strengthen our affiliative nervous system: It may serve to keep the fight-or-flight and pleasure-reward systems in check. This is important, as our tendency toward either perpetual red alert, overactive reward seeking (addictions, for example), or both can sometimes spiral out of control. If you're content with yourself and others, then you are not only less driven to worry excessively about threat but also less given to strive compulsively for the next great thrill (like the impulsive behavior that fuels addiction), or inhale a hamburger when you're stressed or unhappy. An overactive fight-or-flight network produces hypervigilance and anxiety, which is detrimental to health. Excessive reward-seeking behavior can also harm health. An overactive reward system may manifest in more subtle ways, such as workaholism, that are tougher for us to recognize, especially as we live in a culture that champions long and almost ridiculous work hours. We generally think of accomplishment of any kind as a good thing, but there can be a cost to excessive striving, as shown by research demonstrating higher mortality among people who work the longest hours. (This is a body of literature that I prefer not to read in too much detail, because I am one of those people!) Avoiding threats and seeking rewards are part of survival, but only when activated in moderation. When we cultivate our affiliative network and learn to enjoy simply being present — with ourselves and with others — we offer ourselves a much-needed break from our usual routines.

How does this soothing system work in tandem with its sister systems? First, recall from chapter 1 that negative self-talk not only gets us psychologically agitated, but puts our body in a state of fight-or-flight, which means full steam ahead from the perspective of our neurologic, cardiovascular, immune, and endocrine (glandular) systems. This is necessary to get us through certain dire situations, such as running away from a charging elephant (I did not tell you about *that* experience, which I had in Botswana). But being on edge day in and day out — i.e., sitting in your office or your living room ruminating about some threat, perceived or real — can have the same effect, and is harmful to your body. That much you've already heard from me. What Chris and his colleagues are adding to this conversation is that when we look upon ourselves with the warmth of self-compassion, we take ourselves out of red alert and literally soothe ourselves, or allow ourselves to be soothed by others.

It's ironic, but for all the evolutionary importance of our affiliative network during our first years of life, as we grow, our motivations tend to become overshadowed by our continued practice of detecting and evading threat on the one hand and striving for resources on the other. In short, unless we deliberately nurture our affiliative circuit, it gets weaker and weaker, and our ability to generate the state of deep contentment with ourselves and others in effect atrophies like an old, unused muscle. When this happens, our inner dialogue can become overly harsh. "For many of us," Chris says, grimacing, "this conversation is not too pretty." We all know this intuitively, having heard our own voice dish out insults like, "I'm weak" or "I'm so stupid," or "Why can't I shake these feelings? Why can't I get through this? *What's wrong with me?*"

This same inner voice may comment relentlessly on our performance, continually finding fault and holding us back from making any real behavioral headway: "I can't stick to my [exercise, dietary, drug rehab, counseling, fill in the blank] program because I have no willpower, and I never get things done." In my case, I was too close to my own voice to be able to hear it accurately, until one day when I overheard my older daughter harshly scolding my younger one. I was taken aback, because I recognized myself in that tongue lashing — both as the lasher and as the (self-) lashed. I immediately thought, "I sound like that to them, don't I?" and "Hey, I've heard that same voice talking to me!" I walked over to my kids and told them what had just gone through my mind. They stopped arguing and looked at me with such wide eyes that I could feel myself tearing up. In their faces I saw the little person in me who cringed at that voice, and who longed to hear kindness.

To put this process in the CBT terms we discussed in chapter 4, our cognitive distortions are all too often running the show, and Chris, an outlook guide for decades, has heard them all from his clients. He points out the overarching problem as having a high degree of inner criticism, which is always distorted, even for those of us (which means all of us) who have truly messed up in some way at one time or another: "Now, how can you have a reasonably happy, peaceful life if you're hearing this crap in your head all the time?" These continuous messages of doubt, fear, skepticism, and in some cases outright denigration wear us down like water pounding rocks, and cloud our outlook with "I can't." This is in contrast to what Chris terms *discernment* — our ability to objectively view ourselves and our situation without breaking ourselves down. Discernment is the cornerstone of our relationship with ourselves and with others, because it highlights the areas that need to be improved. But how do we distinguish being discerning from being self-critical? I have been practicing compassion exercises for years, and honestly, I still sometimes have trouble in this gray zone. Here is an example from my own life, which I discussed with Chris to get his professional opinion.

I was recently with my husband and what looked like a hundred other people corralled behind a busy Panera lunch counter. As I waited for our order, I watched a young mother across the room hold her baby as she stood with another woman who appeared to be the baby's nanny, ready to stroll the child away. The mother cradled it fiercely, as if she had to squeeze a day's worth of hugs into that narrow and frenetic window. Having already gone through eleven years of relentless work schedules and too-little time with my kids, I felt that mother's desperation with overwhelming pangs of longing to hold my own tiny warm bundle. My first automatic thought was that I should have stayed home to raise my kids full-time. (This would have made a successful medical research career exceedingly difficult, which is why I elected not to do it in the first place.) My second automatic thought was that I was putting my children through the same situation I had experienced as a little girl, pining for my father. (After my parents divorced he gave up teaching English, stopped writing, moved to California, and became a brakeman with the Southern Pacific railroad, which took him out into the Mojave Desert for days at a time.) At the thought of this I teared up right in the midst of the customer mob.

The interesting part about this whole experience, which lasted only a few minutes, was that even while it was happening, I knew I was filling in all kinds of missing data with my own beliefs — the *B* in the ABCs that we discussed in chapter 4. I tried to console myself by thinking that maybe the mother was spending plenty of time with her baby, and that I was jumping to conclusions. I went on to try and convince myself that my own children didn't miss me and my husband on nights and weekends as much as I thought they did. But I knew that wasn't true because now, as six- and eleven-year-old talkers, they had told us repeatedly that they wanted us to be home more. In short, none of those mental gymnastics stopped me from pronouncing myself guilty as charged, and I felt too sick to eat my soup and baguette.

I related all this to my husband, who quickly reoriented me with a quote from Carl Jung, which we have often used to steady each other, and which essentially says that nothing affects children more than the "unlived life" of the parents. For me, both Jung and my husband were right. Had I not continued to work in my current capacity, the lack of fulfillment would undoubtedly have spilled over in unhealthy ways and affected my kids. "You can't keep judging yourself for that," my husband told me. "You're only considering the consequences to the path you chose, and you're assuming there wouldn't be any consequences to the path you didn't choose, and you can't assume that." He reminded me how much we do prioritize our kids, even with the long work hours. And then I noticed the quality of my inner conversation shift to a softer, more inviting voice: "Spend just a few more hours a week with the girls — at the park, painting toenails, whatever." In contrast to my self-critical voice a few minutes earlier, I now recognized the voice of discernment. This was advice I needed to follow. I was still working too much and I knew it, which may be why I had such a strong emotional reaction to the mother with her baby. Feeling a little more relaxed now, my hunger returned. Over lunch I resolved to set up additional daily time and activities with my kids.

Chris made a couple of key points about

my experience. The first is that when we discern something, we hold the problem in a broader context. I saw that my conflict wasn't all about my personal failure as a mom, but rather part of what Chris describes as a "broader, multidimensional conversation. Seeing the broader context has the element of 'wisdom.' What's wisdom? Perhaps understanding the complexity of the situation and seeing your way through." A posthumous reminder from Carl Jung (reaching out through language and culture!) set my situation in context: Lots of people struggle with the unlived life, or aspects of it, one way or another. The second point was that discernment feels different than self-criticism. Listening to my self-critical voice by the deli counter literally turned my stomach, a discomfort that abated only once I was able to hear a kinder, gentler voice from my husband and from myself. "Self-criticism depletes our energy and discernment strengthens us in a quiet way," Chris says. "Discernment is how a wise friend would speak with us, and criticism is how an angry person addresses us. There is a sense of warmth and care in a discerning conversation, and coldness in a critical one."

Some of us may resist self-compassion

because we feel we do not deserve it. Now here's the $64,000 question, if you're old enough to catch that reference. What if we believe that we *are* "deserving" of harsh criticism because we *are* cowardly, weak, or otherwise awful? Obviously, those labels are always subjective and therefore subject to major cognitive distortions. Nevertheless, Chris considers such cases as follows: Everyone has weaknesses and everyone has done something wrong — that's life. I agree. This universal truth is famously captured in the parable of Jesus and the alleged adulteress, which applies to you whether you are religious or not: No one met criteria to cast the first stone. Two thousand years later, nothing has changed in that department. Especially if we have seriously transgressed, Chris invites us to adopt a self-compassionate attitude, just like a mom or dad who is trying to help a wayward child: "As a parent, is it helpful to attack a child's personality, or is it better to direct attention to unskillful or unwholesome behaviors in a supportive, collaborative way?"

Some of us may also resist self-kindness and compassion because we believe it is "wussy" or "soft." Chris has fielded many concerns from people who ask, "Will I lower my standard if I stop criticizing myself, and never improve?" The answer is a definitive "No." Whenever appropriate, we can still discern that change is needed and act accordingly. The key is in *how* we deliver that message to ourselves. Self-compassion and the deep sense of self-worth that it fosters are at the very foundation of our physical and mental health. People with a high degree of self-compassion, like those who are highly optimistic, experience greater psychological well-being and tend to practice health-promoting behaviors. And do we know anything about how to actually cultivate greater self-compassion? Yes. Chris and his colleague Dr. Kristen Neff, of the University of Texas at Austin (the main author of the Self-Compassion Scale, which you completed in chapter 3), have codeveloped the Mindful Self-Compassion program, an eight-week intervention to teach children and adults how to relate to themselves and their failures with understanding and kindness. They recently published a pilot randomized controlled trial demonstrating that people who have gone through the Mindful Self-Compassion program, relative to those in a wait-listed control group, showed greater gains in mindfulness, self-compassion, compassion toward others, and general satisfaction with their lives.

People in the mindful self-compassion group also experienced decreases in anxiety, depression, and stress. At the end of this section I've included an exercise from the program so you can start practicing self-compassion ASAP!

Chris works with people every day who are self-critical to the point where it interferes with whatever they may try to accomplish. "We have people who are just full of shame, who feel completely unworthy, who have been traumatized — I mean, just a broad, broad spectrum of people for whom self-kindness is a horrifying, terrifying thing. But I look at that not as a problem, but as the process." He recalls watching a video about teaching mindfulness to Vietnam veterans, and hearing the words of one veteran who was learning the process of mindfulness: "I've been calling myself 'traitor' ever since I left my buddy who got blown up, you know, and I've been carrying his picture in my pocket for forty years." Chris has one answer for such dark outlook places: "It's time to change the conversation."

In the Mindful Self-Compassion program, people are encouraged to cast away their fears of vulnerability and cut themselves some slack, however small that slack may be at first. Remember incremental optimism from chapter 2? Even small shifts can bring big results. As you might have guessed, the first step is to open our eyes and ears to our inner conversation. Like many outlook guides, Chris uses combinations of the techniques I introduced in chapter 4 — with an emphasis on mindfulness — to help people achieve this. Next he adds an interesting twist to the process by emphasizing "an attitude *within* awareness — in other words, loving awareness, tender awareness, gentle awareness, warm awareness. The *quality* of the awareness is actually more important and more predictive of positive outcomes, such as improvement in feelings of anxiety and depression."

Otherwise, highly focused awareness can be almost as uncomfortable as the experience of feeling bad — essentially when you are feeling bad about feeling bad. This is what Buddhists refer to as "the second arrow." You get hit with one arrow — an argument, an accident, a death, something painful and perhaps unexpected, however large or small — then let the ensuing rage, shock, fear, or guilt wound you over and over as you relive the experience and berate yourself for incompetently managing it. While an acute reaction to pain is normal and healthy, the problems start when those arrows keep flying, sometimes nonstop, sometimes for years.

Chris teaches clients to bring warmth and self-caring to their inner awareness, which acts as a kind of cease-fire so the healing can begin. The full Mindful Self-Compassion program developed by Chris and Kristin makes use of many exercises. The following is an abridged and para-phrased version.

Exercise: Cultivating Self-Compassion

Sit in an upright and comfortable position. You may close your eyes or leave them open. Take a few breaths to settle in and focus on the present moment.

Place your hand on your heart as a physical reminder to be kind to yourself.

Bring your attention inside your body and feel its pulsation, including the rhythm of your breathing and heartbeat.

Begin to notice physical sensations of stress that you're holding in your body,

270

and where they are (jaw, neck, abdomen, etc.).

Next, begin to notice any emotional stress — feelings of worry, such as anxiety about the future or uneasiness about the past. Understand that every human body bears stress and worry throughout the day.

Now make an offering of goodwill to yourself, because of the stress that you're holding in your body, as we all hold stress in our bodies from morning till night. Gently and slowly, tell yourself the following: "May I be safe. May I be peaceful. May I be kind to myself. May I accept myself as I am." Feel free to choose any phrases that might work better for you — words that are just what you need to hear in this moment. See if you can give yourself that gift.

Difficult emotions will naturally arise. If you become overwhelmed, you can name the emotion (fear, anger), find where it seems strongest in your body, and breathe into that area to soften it. Alternatively, for emotions that are overpowering, return your attention to your breathing. When you are comfortable, you may return to the preceding phrases.

End with a few breaths, knowing that you can return to the phrases anytime you wish.

Gently open your eyes, stretch your arms and legs, and bring your awareness back to your surroundings.

If the process sounds pretty easy, I'll give you my take, having practiced similar exercises for years. It *can* be easy, but there are many obstacles that tend to arise, such as mind wandering, the urgency to get up and do "more important" things, falling asleep, and, well, that inner voice that pops up to say, "This is silly." The latter can be a particularly tough obstacle arising in those of us with stiff upper lips. To get past it, Chris encourages people to imagine they are addressing themselves as young children, or perhaps a sick relative or friend, or even their fallen brothers (and sisters) in arms. Then speak from that place of love, respect, and connection. Just as I noted earlier for the larger process of cultivating our outlook, it is sometimes easier to cultivate compassion when we focus on our loved ones. We also need to remember that there are consequences to not cutting ourselves some slack. Not only does self-criticism feel bad; it can hinder our road to good health. Finally, it's important to remember that just like most medicines and healthy behaviors, it's important to give yourself "doses" of self-compassion on most days, if not several times a day.

"SUSAN": THE POWER OF EMPATHY

Next I'll introduce you to a guide who could be your next door neighbor. I call her Susan, a pseudonym I've given to protect her identity and the identities of her clientele, all of whom are ten and under. She is a living embodiment of the very kindness Dr. Germer and colleagues advocate — the trump card evolution has dealt us to be able to experience a deep sense of peace and safety. Susan is a teacher's aide in a Title I school set within a financially and socially depressed district on the West Coast. Only about one in ten kids pay for their lunch; the rest qualify for state and federal aid programs.

Not infrequently, the school goes into lockdown status (when no one is allowed in or out of the building), an event often prompted by unstable parent situations and involving the police. As you can imagine, the chaotic environments that many of these kids grow up in are not conducive to making them feel safe. Yet children depend on a sense of security for their growth and survival, and Susan, whose compassion cup is overflowing, pours as much as possible into as many little people as she can.

Having worked in this capacity for over twenty years, she has been charged with assisting kids who aren't able to manage in the regular classroom because they have fallen too far behind — she effectively functions as the safety net below the safety net. From the small room she shares with several other educators, Susan and her colleagues make it their daily priority to provide a safe haven that also happens to be full of amazing and cool things to learn. Often those things stem from the natural world, given that these people live enviably close to some of the most beautiful coastline on earth. What Susan has seen over the years is something we all know, but that we also tend to forget: Other people have much more going on than we can see, and a kid's resistance to learning doesn't necessarily mean he isn't capable or willing to try. But Susan does not forget. "These poor kids — they didn't ask to be thrown into such circumstances. Some of the stuff that they go through would keep any of us from being able to concentrate."

Susan talks about Karl, a third-grader who was living out of his mother's car and having trouble with the other kids at school for a number of reasons, which included his lack of access to a shower on days when his family couldn't get into a shelter. Understandably, he didn't smell very good. Compounding matters, Karl, who had the reading level of a first-grader, was far behind his classmates, and had become so anxious about being called on that he couldn't sit and pay attention in a regular classroom. With great sensitivity, Susan and her colleagues helped him with his hygiene, and then set about the more difficult task of equipping Karl with some skills to focus on his reading and math. After a few days of trial and error, Susan found out that he liked music, and started each session with a few minutes of listening to a calming piece, telling him, "Karl, this is something you can do when you're feeling upset — you can put your headphones on, and then once you're feeling a little better, the headphones come off and you open your book." The plan worked. Susan focused his reading material on things that he loved, like orca whales, and used this to motivate Karl to read, type, and write. Over time, he came into her classroom and began reading, unprompted.

Susan is about as polite and proper as they come — but there is one thing that she cannot tolerate: seeing adults (and even other kids) passing judgment on her students before bothering to find out the circumstances. "If you work with these little guys one-on-one, it really can change the way they see things. Sometimes I get frustrated, when I see other adults — parents, teachers, whoever — crack down on the kids. On the one hand, I can understand why the adults would be upset. They are trying to do their job, maybe trying to run a classroom of twenty-five or thirty kids as smoothly as possible, and then when one child repeatedly exhibits disruptive behavior, it's easy to see how they may label that child as a 'problem,' and conclude that he or she just needs to 'buck up.' On the other hand, if you just take the time to ask that child what's going on . . . 'What happened the night before? Did you get enough sleep? Did you eat dinner last night?' You see how some of the problems these kids are facing aren't going away by 'bucking up.' You've got to ask yourself — have you walked in their shoes? Do you know what some of them are really going through?"

So what kinds of things are happening to these kids? Things that none of us would ever want for our kids or ourselves. Susan lists just a few. "The police come and arrest the dad, or older brother or sister. Sometimes there are serious arguments in the home, with a lot of screaming, even physical violence. Sometimes the parents have alcohol and drug problems. Obviously, none of this makes the kids feel safe." Susan remembers one time when the parents of a first-grader left him home alone all night. "They just never showed up at all, and the child had to get himself to sleep and ready for school the next day." How can a six- or seven-year-old sit and do math problems after such wrenching hardships? Susan answers candidly: "They can't." As might be expected, some children are transitioned by the state into foster care, but Susan is quick to note that this is not a blame game. "A lot of these parents are just trying to survive. Many are unemployed, many are trying to find work." The school does help them with paperwork to qualify for social programs to help stabilize the family. "You can only stay in those shelters for so many days, and then you have to move. In some of the shelters, the boys aren't able to stay with their moms, and are taken to a separate facility somewhere else in the city. I'd almost rather live in my car than be separated from my kids in those circumstances."

Susan had her own protracted experience as a child struggling to learn in school. Interestingly, her very first Point A (original attitude latitude) was reasonably positive and carefree. She was the youngest of five children, and for the first few years of her life her parents kept a small but solid home on her father's salary at a local lumber mill. Her parents talked of plans to build a larger house in a nicer area of town, along with other expectations of good things to come. That all changed when Susan's father died suddenly just before her third birthday, and his untimely death in an era before life insurance was common drove them into dire financial straits. Her mother did not receive any financial support from her extended family, which meant Susan's older brothers and sisters, in high school at the time, had to work to make ends meet. The change also set the stage for ridicule at school, where the kids "made fun of me because I didn't have a dad."

Susan's mother, whom she remembers as an emotional rock, was not able to help much with Susan's studies, because she now had to work so many evening hours that she was simply not available. When her mother finally remarried, it solved the "no dad" problem, but did nothing to plug the educational mentorship hole. Sadly, having been orphaned and raised on a work farm, her step-dad had barely seen the inside of an eighth-grade classroom, so it was not surprising that he wasn't able to help sufficiently with her homework. Susan was caught in a downward spiral.

And then the first of several people whom she now credits with helping her grow up to be the person she is today arrived on the scene. Brian, a long-time friend of the family and pharmacy school student who had recently moved back into town, offered to tutor her with the limited time he had available. It marked the beginning of her turning point — here was someone who actually had the education and the ability to uplift her spirits as he taught her, making jokes and laughing to lighten the mood. "He didn't put me down if I didn't understand something. He knew I was struggling." His tutoring, and the sense of confidence it gave her, got Susan through fifth grade. She realized she was now starting to see the possibility of future success. Brian had unwittingly played the role of an outlook guide. In such examples we see how we can all guide others' outlook — perhaps without even knowing it. What matters is that we are helping others as we do what we do.

Then something truly extraordinary happened. Her seventh-grade homeroom teacher, whom she remembers as a "tall, thin, kind woman," sized up Susan on day one and locked on to her academic needs with the fierce protectiveness of a mother bear. "She spent extra time with me every day for a year," Susan says, still shaking her head in disbelief and gratitude that a stranger could alter her life course so profoundly. "She gave me help and encouraged me. She just worked with me from ground zero. And even when I struggled, she would say, 'Susan, it's OK, you're going to get it. No problem.' She took me from the lowest spelling group to the highest spelling group. She took me from someone who was getting C's and D's to someone who was getting straight A's. She gave me hope. Just one person can make that big a difference in another person's life." That single devoted teacher transformed Susan's outlook to get excited about learning, but more important, the experience showed her a path to do the same for others, the path she now walks every day.

As part of her college studies in psychology, Susan interned as a counselor at a shelter for battered women and their children, before landing a position as a welfare caseworker, which she found absolutely fulfilling. "Our unit worked with those families — those clients that either needed to get their GED or go to a one- or two-year program." She would send out monthly questionnaires, and then based on the data clients provided, "I would target those who needed extra help. They would send me their grades, and I'd have to make sure that they had their scholarships, or their way of paying for the program." She also made frequent phone calls to her five hundred clients. "They knew that they had access to me any time of day in the office." She relished her job for three years, but even with the satisfaction of knowing she was helping entire families through the work she was doing, she longed to work directly with kids, perhaps because of her own experiences earlier in life. So when a job opened up as an educational assistant in a nearby school district, she jumped at the chance.

As if she needed any more inspiration to get up in the morning, Susan's determination was only fortified after she narrowly survived a horrific car accident that killed two of her friends and left her permanently injured. It started with the bad decision to take a ride with a friend who wanted to show off his new sports car. Unbeknownst to Susan, he was also an alcoholic who already had several DUIs under his belt. They flew through an intersection against a flashing red light and were T-boned by a station wagon, sending them hurtling into the porch of a nearby house and knocking it a foot off the foundation. Hearing the crash, the inhabitants of the house came out and threw sheets on all four motionless and bloodied passengers, whom they took for dead. "I remember waking up and being really irate," Susan recalls. "I figured we had gone off the road. I thought everyone else had already gotten out of the car and left me there. It was only when I tried to move and couldn't that I realized, 'Whoa, I'm in trouble.' And then I heard voices saying, 'Oh my God, she's alive!' "

In fact, the gearshift had gone through her pelvic bone, fracturing it in six places, and she had broken her jaw. As fortune would have it, the first people on the scene (after the house owners) were a registered nurse and a paramedic. They called ahead to the nearest ER, which, luckily for her, already had a fully mobilized trauma team. After a prolonged ICU stay and multiple surgeries, she finally made it out to the regular hospital floor in traction, followed by weeks of rehab.

And then she met another outlook guide — a physical therapist who took care of many of the premier athletes in town. "She was regarded as one of the best in her field," Susan said. "She would stand me out in the middle of the floor and then take away my walker and say, 'Susan, you can either take a step, or you can stay there all day. It's entirely up to you. Walk, and you're going to be able to walk out of here to the rest of your life.'" Susan remembers thinking, "If she's willing to help me recover, then the least I can do is to give it a whirl." The tough love paid off, and she is now able to walk and do most things that she loves, including help her students realize their potential. "I want to make a difference in people's lives. I am here for a reason." She has daily pain in her hip and left lower extremity — pain that she interprets as nothing other than a reminder that she is lucky to be alive.

Susan overcame many odds and could have easily given in to a pessimistic or cynical outlook. How many people would *you* put your trust in after losing your father and having your emotional wounds salted daily by the jeers of classmates? And what about driving anywhere after that motor vehicle accident — how long would it take *you* to get behind a wheel again? (She began driving several months after completing physical therapy.) She could easily have stayed in fight-or-flight mode in any of these situations, revving her red-alert engines ad infinitum and numbing herself with drugs, alcohol, or bad relationships. But she didn't, in part because of the outlook guides that had landed in her life, whom she listened to and trusted, and in part because of her own empathy toward others that she recognized in herself "even since I was a little child." She also remained open to learning new things and trying new ways of problem solving, character traits that allowed her to fully accept the help that she was offered. Throughout everything, she showed trust and friendliness (what psychologists term "agreeableness"), making her a very easy person to take care of.

We haven't spent much time discussing agreeableness — another Big Five trait — primarily because it has not received as much attention in the health and aging research. People who are more agreeable tend to have less delinquency. They also adapt better after a medical illness or setback. (Agreeableness does not mean putting others' needs over and above our own. Rather, it describes our capacity to take interest in and empathize with others.) Practically speaking, agreeable people also may be easier to help — just as I found out with my heart surgeon, who upon seeing my complete willingness to seek his advice and enthusiasm to follow it, took me under his wing and helped me long after my scars had healed. Something I didn't tell you earlier is that four years after my surgery, as a senior medical student, I did what's called a "rotation" with him on the cardiovascular surgery service for several weeks, and got the chance to work with the very same OR team that had handled my case. Three years after that, Dr. Karp filled in for my late father and walked me down the aisle at my wedding. Eight years later, when he and his wife died in an automobile accident in the Loire Valley in France, it was like losing family.

Agreeableness is a key ingredient to social support and social bonding. Perhaps Susan's agreeableness, along with her deeper determination to lend a hand, formed the bedrock of her resilience, resulting in a truly superstar ability to affiliate with others — drawing as much comfort *from* them as she returned *to* them — a feature that she has carried forward in her current profession, where she continues to be nourished by, and to nourish, her students. Outlook guides are all around us, leading by example and directly lending a hand. In the next chapter we'll see how we may rely on them even more when our physical or mental health falters.

7

LOOKING UP IS ESPECIALLY IMPORTANT WHEN YOU'RE "DOWN"

Looking up is a practice that is crucial for everyone, but especially for people who are weighed down with physical and mental health problems. For example, in our research of older women, my colleagues and I have found that as the number of cardiovascular risk factors goes up, so does the risk gap between optimists and pessimists. In other words, among healthy people without any major risk factors, optimists and pessimists die at about the same rate. But among people with one major risk factor (such as diabetes), pessimists have higher death rates, and this trend amplifies in people as they become increasingly burdened with cardiovascular disease risk factors. We saw a similar trend for cynical hostility, the deep-seated mistrust of people: The difference in the risk of death between someone with high cynical hostility versus someone with low cynical hostility gets bigger as the number of cardiovascular risk factors goes up. In plain terms, this means that the more risk factors you have, the more important your outlook is for health and longevity. In this same study, we examined five major cardiovascular disease risk factors (which you'll recall from our discussion of ideal cardiac health in chapter 1) — high blood pressure, high cholesterol, diabetes, obesity, and smoking — and divided women into categories based on how many of these risk factors they had. In this sample of almost one hundred thousand postmenopausal women, 23 percent had no risk factors and 8 percent had three or more risk factors.

Plenty of research shows that traditional risk factor burden, independent of a person's outlook, strongly predicts future cardiovascular disease (meaning heart attack, stroke, peripheral vascular disease) and death from these causes. In my study it was no different: Women with healthier risk factor profiles had the lowest rates of death, while those with more risk factors had higher rates of death. As you might expect by now, the optimists in my study tended to have fewer risk factors than pessimists: Thirty-two percent of optimists were risk factor–free, while only 22 percent had three or more risk factors. (The rest had one or two risk factors.) The trend was almost exactly opposite for pessimists, who were much more likely to be burdened by more cardiovascular disease risk factors. Now, here is the really interesting part. In women with one risk factor, pessimists were 27 percent more likely than optimists to die. In contrast, among women who had three or more cardiovascular risk factors, pessimists were 73 percent more likely than optimists to die during that same period. For cynical hostility, among women with one risk factor, those with high cynical hostility were 21 percent more likely to die. But among women with three or more risk factors, those with high cynical hostility were 63 percent more likely to die.

So why should the magnitude of the effect of outlook — whether we are talking about pessimism, cynical hostility, or other traits — be different for people who are more heavily burdened by cardiovascular risk factors? Why should outlook matter more for people who are medically "down"? A big part of the answer, as we've seen, is that our outlook naturally influences the way we care for ourselves. Thus the associated benefits of looking up have to do with the fact that a brighter disposition goes hand in hand with better self-care and making healthier choices. Expecting good things to come, optimists may envision better health and work toward that goal by taking medication, exercising, and following doctor's orders.

Alternatively, people with a high degree of pessimism may shun self-care altogether if they view it as pointless. Self-care is important for anyone, but it is even more critical for people who have multiple health risk factors, because the consequences of not tending to those risk factors become rapidly apparent. As I'll show you, the fatalistic diabetic who doesn't really believe taking his medication will make a difference one way or the other is bound to have a heart attack quicker than the fatalistic nondiabetic person, all other aspects of their health being equal. I want to emphasize that this fatalism is not necessarily due to depression — it also occurs in people who do not have mental health problems. A fatalistic or otherwise negatively valenced mind-set is not considered a disease, but as we've seen so far, it can misguide us toward wretched states of physical health.

THE CASE OF JASON

Jason was a man with type 1 diabetes in his early twenties who became my hospital patient three times in the same month for life-threatening diabetic ketoacidosis (or DKA for short), a condition in which lack of insulin leads to acidification of the blood and impending death. Type 1 diabetics are at particularly high risk for DKA since they are dependent on doses of medically prepared insulin, usually via injection. If the body doesn't get enough insulin, it must shift biochemical gears to produce enough energy for basic metabolism, and this emergency pathway yields a high acid load, which soon overwhelms the buffering capacity of the lungs and kidneys. When blood pH falls far enough, all organ systems begin to shut down unless medical care is rendered to correct the imbalance.

With the exception of episodes brought on by severe infection, heart attack, or other major medical illness, DKA is mostly preventable by taking insulin and following a healthy lifestyle. This is where Jason's attitude was hampering his chances of making it to the next week, let alone to a ripe old age. His identical twin brother was unaffected by diabetes, and Jason felt that he had been dealt an unfair hand. He deeply resented the need to follow a strict diet and take medication. Consequently, he did neither, which set the stage for his repeated bouts of DKA.

When he was admitted twice in about a week for the same problems, I caught on to his attitude and we had our first meaningful conversation — beyond medication, carbonated drinks, and other shoulds and shouldn'ts. One day after rounds I went into his room by myself, without the larger team of residents and students, and sat down to talk to him. That was when he told me in so many words about his anger and fear about the diabetes, which, in sharp contrast to his brother's health, seemed more menacing every day. Besides, he revealed, he didn't expect to live long anyway. But in that same conversation, he also volunteered that he liked writing and performing his own songs, and frequented a local recording studio. I caught that spark and tried to fan it using some of the motivational interviewing techniques we learned in chapter 4.

I told him that while I didn't have type 1 diabetes, I did understand what it felt like to be born into less-than-ideal medical circumstances (expressing empathy). I also pointed out the obvious fact that avoiding his diabetes was only hurting him more by keeping him from his music (developing discrepancy between his current path and the path he wanted to take). "I know," he said, but then shrugged it off. I had to figure out a way to convince him that his current mind-set of expecting the worst was only fulfilling his prophecy of early death. Wanting to make sure he knew he had a future, I emphasized that I and other doctors treated plenty of type 1 diabetics who were much older than he was, and that he was capable of living a long and healthy life as a composer, singer, and DJ. He at last began to look at me, and I could tell he was listening. As before, his medical condition improved and he was discharged.

When he rolled up to the medical floor about a week and a half later with a third episode of DKA, I didn't let him end our conversation so easily. "Listen, Jason. I need to know what's going on." Over the next few minutes I learned that his brother, who already had a job and a wife, was now having a baby. While he was happy for his brother and excited about being an uncle, his own self-worth had plummeted as he succumbed to fears that he would never be able to achieve these life goals. Such self-destructive behavior is striking, but I should point out that noncompliance with medical care does not necessarily equal depression or mental incompetence. He had neither of these, as I confirmed on the third admission with a formal psychiatric evaluation.

One day while rounding alone, I asked him as plainly as I could, "What do you want out of your life?" Part of the technique of developing discrepancy is describing in the clearest terms possible what you really want — your best case scenario — and then honestly assessing whether what you're doing now is likely to get you there. But hope takes courage, and sometimes even describing one's dreams out loud may seem like a daunting task. So I was not surprised when he didn't answer me right away, and I allowed the ensuing silence to linger a moment before continuing, "Do you plan to develop your music career? Do you want to have a family?" Again, silence. Finally he told me, "I guess I never really thought about it." As we talked more, I learned he actually did think about the future often but his thoughts were so focused on the misconception that his illness was strangling any hope of accomplishment (an understandably scary prospect) that he quickly pushed them out of his mind whenever possible. He had never felt comfortable talking about this with his family or friends, and had never seen a counselor.

Our team, whom he had come to know fairly well over the prior weeks, kept working with Jason and gradually he opened up even further. He agreed to try out a diabetes support group. Interestingly, the person who had perhaps the greatest impact on Jason's turnaround was his hospital roommate, an engaging diabetic old-timer who was in for a heart failure exacerbation. One afternoon I was washing my hands in the hallway right outside their room and overheard the roommate giving Jason some sound advice: "You need to preserve your health, kid! You've got your whole life to live. How are you gonna do your music if you're in the hospital all the time?" The roommate went on to relate how even in his own current state, his medications gave him the chance to do the things he loved, like walk his dog to the park and get out of the house to visit with friends. Intrigued, I stayed at the sink as long as I could. I heard Jason answering him affirmatively, and I could tell by the strength and tone of his voice that something major had clicked. By the time Jason was ready for discharge a few days later, he was not only telling the nurses how he wanted to keep singing and get a girlfriend, but he was even administering his own insulin. So began an evolution of Jason's outlook from fatalistic apathy to mustering enough courage to hope for a few simple life goals and start working toward them. Had Jason not accepted the recommendations to examine his outlook and speed up his "travel" plans when he did, he would have remained at very high risk of more diabetic complications and premature death.

POINT A TO POINT B: EVEN SMALL DIFFERENCES IN OUTLOOK MATTER FOR HEALTHY AGING

As you know by now, people don't typically revolutionize their attitude overnight. In addition to taking things slowly, it's important that we set reasonable goals so that we don't psych ourselves out or bite off more than we can chew, feel like failures, and then never try again. Fortunately, research shows that even a one-point difference in attitude latitude, as measured by the LOT-R, translates into clinically important differences in the risk of disease and death. My colleagues and I found in our study of older women that being one point more pessimistic translated into a 2 percent higher risk of heart disease and a 4 percent higher risk of death from any cause. Considering that an optimist and a pessimist are typically at least

296

four to five points apart on the scale depending on the population studied, those risks can really add up.

It's important to understand that this particular study did not test for *change* in optimism over time, because most people only provided information on how optimistic their Point A was, and were not asked to repeat the questionnaire, probably because, as we discussed earlier, optimism and other aspects of outlook have long been considered fairly static after early adulthood. Only recently has the notion of actively cultivating outlook for the benefit of health started to gain more traction. While my study did not measure the women's change in optimism over time, it did measure their health risk over a decade, so at the very least we can compare people who had small differences in their Point A to start with and see that this small difference corresponded to a big difference in health risk down the road.

One difficulty in trying to link research findings (e.g., from my study) to clinical examples (the case of Jason) is that we don't have all the data in either situation. For instance, I didn't administer any psychological questionnaires to Jason during his hospital stays in order to gauge his outlook trek from Point A to Point B. But his attitudinal shifts, which to me and other people on his medical team were unmistakable, led to noticeable differences in his behavior over the course of that remarkable month. As you know, behavior is a huge driver of your life span and your health span. If I had to estimate based on my knowledge of the LOT-R, I would venture that Jason shifted no more than a point or two toward greater hopefulness for the future, but it had quite an effect on his mind and body. You can probably think of someone in your life (maybe it's you) whose outlook has shifted slightly from Point A to Point B, with corresponding changes in conduct — taking medication, starting an exercise program, cutting down on tobacco use, or something else, all of which are known to promote healthy aging.

Jason's case is a very compelling argument for self-care, whether you have no health risk factors or ten. I find it useful to combine data from such illustrative individuals with epidemiologic research on entire populations, in which the sheer numbers speak for themselves. As you read on, I invite you to think about where you fall on the risk factor spectrum and consider what outlook travel steps you could take to improve your situation healthwise. You can also do this exercise by keeping in mind someone you care about.

Let's revisit the data from the large 2012 study on lifetime risks of cardiovascular disease that I introduced in chapter 2. The study combined data from eighteen studies involving more than 250,000 men and women age 45 to 75 (and of different races) to determine the lifetime risk of cardiovascular disease based on whether people had optimal cardiovascular disease profiles. The profile is very similar to the "ideal cardiac health" that I introduced in chapter 1.

The investigators considered five categories of risk, ranging from all risk factors optimal (low risk) to having two or more major risk factors (high risk). They used the term *lifetime risk* to refer to the chances of getting cardiovascular disease or dying from it by age 80 (for those who started the study at age 45 or 55) or by age 90 (for those who started at age 65 or 75). If you're wondering where Jason might fit into these data, consider that he was half the age of the youngest person in the study, but was still at relatively high risk of cardiovascular disease and death because his diabetes had been so poorly controlled for so long. So his risk actually approached that of someone much older.

Across all ages, people with fewer risk factors had much lower lifetime rates of cardiovascular disease events and death than those with more risk factors. I mentioned this concept earlier, but showing the numbers really drives home the point. For example, only about 2 percent of 45-year-olds in the lowest risk category suffered a heart attack or died from coronary heart disease by age 80, compared with 42 percent of those in the highest risk category! Among 75-year-olds, only 9 percent of those with optimal cardiovascular risk profiles (lowest risk) had a heart attack or died from coronary heart disease by age 90, compared to 35 percent of those with two or more major risk factors (highest risk).

You can see why avoiding these risk factors in the first place and managing them when they do arise is so key to healthy aging, and why you should use your outlook — and any other tool in your toolbox — on your own behalf.

NUANCES OF OUTLOOK TRAVEL: IS IT MORE IMPORTANT TO BE POSITIVE OR TO NOT BE NEGATIVE?

Jason was lucky enough to realize, if somewhat belatedly, that his pessimistic Point A was threatening his life, and also lucky enough to encounter his prescient room-mate and other outlook guides to help him inch toward a brighter Point B. Whatever his exact mental picture of Point B was, he obviously saw something that he cared about, and his actions showed it. He not only stopped declaring that his future was toast, but he also actively began to look forward to things, including finding a companion. As he lost some of his pessimistic edge, he also began building greater optimism. From my perspective, one of the most interesting research questions is whether high pessimism undermines health, whether high optimism bolsters and protects it, or whether both processes are important. Jason's case, as well as evidence from the existing research, suggests that it's both. Furthermore, optimism may matter more for certain health conditions, while pessimism influences others.

A point of clarification: High pessimism and low optimism are not quite the same thing. High pessimism means actively expecting a dismal future. Low optimism refers to lacking any expectation for a bright future. Before he began to change, Jason's high pessimism (actively expecting negative things to happen) allowed him to ignore his body and fulfill his self-projections of poor health, and his low optimism (not expecting good things to happen) kept him from generating excitement about his future. The disturbing fact that he had "never really thought about it" reminded me of how Dr. Kapoor described many people around him in his youth who were not oriented toward their future: "When you don't think about it, you just float." There are many reasons, including cultural ones, for this orientation, but for Jason it was through avoidance and apathy that he had floated his way into a medically precarious attitude latitude. He was only able to start inching his way out by simultaneously aiming his brain away from the frustration of being a sideshow to his brother's success and toward creating his own success.

Thus, while optimism and pessimism have been traditionally considered as anchors on opposite ends of the same spectrum, in recent years scientists and clinicians alike have begun to consider them as independent traits. This concept can be confusing, so I again turned to Dr. Scheier to clarify matters. When he and his colleagues created the LOT-R, they included three positively worded statements (e.g., "In uncertain times, I expect the best"), which measured optimism, and three negatively worded statements (e.g., "If something can go wrong for me, it will"), which measured pessimism. These optimism and pessimism subscales can be tested separately as predictors of health problems. "The way I try to explain it to people," says Dr. Scheier from his sun-filled office at Carnegie Mellon University, "is this. If I ask you the question, 'Do you expect bad things to happen?' and you say no, then you don't expect bad things to happen. But that may or may not tell me anything about whether you expect *good* things to happen. Because I could then say to you, 'Do you expect good things to happen?' and if you say no, then you don't expect either good or bad things to happen, and that's not an unreasonable kind of view to hold. So just because somebody doesn't expect bad things doesn't necessarily mean they expect good things, either, and vice versa. And so in that way, optimism and pessimism are separable."

This point is very important, because research shows that high pessimism is a major culprit for health all by itself, even independent of a person's level of optimism. High pessimism has been associated with poor health traversing the spectrum of cardiovascular disease risk factors to definitive cardiovascular disease itself. In a large study I conducted with Drs. Scheier, Matthews, Lewis Kuller (whom I'll introduce below), and colleagues in postmenopausal women who were free of cardiovascular disease, high pessimism was the better predictor of heart attack and death. But optimism, independent of a person's level of pessimism, is important for health, too, as I'll show you next.

A HOPEFUL OUTLOOK CAN HELP PULL US OUT OF DEPRESSION

My colleagues Drs. Bruce Rollman and Bea Belnap had recently conducted a clinical trial to treat depression in men and women after coronary artery bypass grafting (CABG), and we collaborated with Drs. Scheier, Matthews, and others to study how optimism and pessimism affected the post-surgical course of these patients. We found that people with high optimism were less likely to be rehospitalized by eight months after surgery. Our study was not designed to understand all of the reasons for this, although people with high optimism were more likely to adhere to their doctor's advice. Two-thirds of the adults were clinically depressed, a common scenario for people with coronary artery disease, and were randomized (like the flip of a coin) to receive one of two treatments for depression. The first treatment was "usual care" from the physician, which as you may know is typically a combination of antidepressant medication and counseling. The other was a collaborative care model in which a dedicated nurse contacted the patients regularly, delivered phone counseling, and coordinated medication prescriptions with the physician when appropriate. Through this study, we uncovered some fascinating aspects of optimism and depression.

Before I go into those, a quick aside: You may be wondering, can an optimist become depressed? Yes! While research shows that over time, optimists are less likely than pessimists to become depressed, they still do, underscoring a critical point: Trait optimism, as measured by the LOT-R, does not necessarily mean the absence of depression, and trait pessimism is not synonymous with depression. While depressed people often endorse hopelessness, depression is a clinical condition that has additional features that may include extreme sadness, suicidality, loss of interest in activities that used to be enjoyable, difficulty sleeping and thinking, etc. Ultimately, though, optimists may have an edge when it comes to getting better, which was the case in our study.

We found that 58 percent of depressed optimists versus only 27 percent of depressed pessimists responded to treatment for their depression. After we controlled for the severity of depression, optimists' depression was about three times as likely as pessimists' to substantially improve. We further learned that symptoms of depression were most likely to improve among the people with high optimism, compared with those with low optimism. Thus, something about optimism — independent of pessimism — predicted this improvement. It may be that the same healthy thought patterns and behaviors that help optimists stay clear of downward mood spirals in the first place actually help them pull themselves back out if they stumble and fall.

It's worth emphasizing that depression, which for too long has been considered a purely mental or psychological affliction, is now understood to be a full-body condition with myriad pathological (biologically harmful) changes taking place underneath the more recognizable outward signs of depressed behavior. Not surprisingly, depressed people tend to behave in unhealthy ways by smoking, hazardous drinking, overeating, and noncompliance with medications and other life-saving medical treatments. If having greater optimism — along with other healthy aspects of our outlook — can help us avoid depression or recover from it more readily when it does affect us, then it is in our own best interest to learn to sprout these seeds wherever possible. A study of whether treatment of mood disorders actually changes optimism, and to what extent, is currently underway.

BUILDING OPTIMISM IN DEPRESSION: THE CASE OF DAVID AND HIS OUTLOOK GUIDE, DR. TOM ALLMON

In chapter 6, I introduced you to several outlook guides not only because they each have an amazing story to tell, but because I believe that while you can accomplish attitudinal change largely on your own, the help of friends, family, professional guides, or all of the above catalyzes this process. It's critical that you have someone in your life (preferably more than one person) who can function in this capacity. In turn, you may play the role of outlook guide for people you know. As we saw with Jason, these guides become especially important when we are medically or psychologically down in the ways that I've described, because during these periods, we have fewer mental and physical resources to keep ourselves on track, even if we're already savvy outlook travelers. This vulnerability is most apparent if we become clinically depressed.

Dr. Tom Allmon is a physician near Portland, Oregon, whom I have known and admired since we met during my first year of clinical practice in primary care. I learned techniques from guides like Tom for a decade before I even began formally studying outlook in relation to health and aging. As a family practitioner, Tom is charged with helping people, and sometimes whole families, with all types of change, like adopting healthier eating habits, getting more exercise, taking necessary medications, quitting smoking, and managing mood disorders, to name a few.

He accomplishes this by drawing on a piece of his cultural heritage that imbues his own outlook: *sisu,* the Finnish term for sustained courage in the face of adversity, an idea that the Finns have historically taken to new heights. No matter how recalcitrant they may be or how hopeless their situation may appear, Tom's patients can count on him to help them get healthy by cultivating their own *sisu.* Tom remembers the case of one particularly memorable fifteen-year-old Native American boy whom we'll call David, who suffered his first bout of major depression a few years after becoming Tom's primary care patient. Tom was able to shepherd him through this difficult year with medical treatment (counseling and antidepressants) and by supporting David's outlook by repeatedly directing his attention back to his own strength of character.

For most of his life, David had been raised by his uncle in the Pacific Northwest because he was estranged from his father, who was severely depressed, addicted to alcohol and drugs, and living a thousand miles away on a reservation in the Southwest. When he started seeing Tom, David was leading a reasonably normal life as a high school student. He studied, did well in school, didn't smoke or drink, and despite being mildly overweight, generally took good care of himself. He had never been diagnosed with depression, but did acknowledge feeling deeply sad about living apart from his father. More than anything else, David wanted a permanent reunion, but due to many factors, including his father's condition, the two had not seen each other for years. Yet David was very forward-looking for his young age, and desperately wanted to help his father and eventually go and live with him. He organized a successful in-person visit, which marked the beginning of reparations. For several months the two were in more frequent contact, and David's father, now in treatment, seemed to be doing better and getting the pieces of his life in order.

Then one day without warning, David's father killed himself, sending David into an emotional tailspin and even prompting hospitalization for depression. Tom remembers those dark days. "He went through a couple of months when he was really in turmoil, and even tried to commit suicide." For a while, it looked as if he was heading toward the same fate as his father, to become yet another sobering Native American statistic. David didn't want to come in to the clinic, but his uncle kept bringing him anyway. Although he was physically sitting in Tom's office, David would just stare at the wall and refuse to engage (not uncommon behavior in severe depression). "For a time there, I just couldn't communicate with him at all," Tom said. "But I kept telling him things, hoping something would stick."

Tom verbally emphasized David's courage. "You are still a very young man — and yet you took it upon yourself to help your father. You made an important effort that shows what a caring individual you are. You have learned that you can't change the outcome in every situation — but what you can do is *try.*" Tom knew David was hearing him because every once in a while David would look up and answer. Gradually, David did start to warm up again, and eventually Tom was even able to counsel him on some of the less pressing but critically important preventive health recommendations. This advice was particularly important for David, whose genes and environment were in cahoots to sentence him not only to repeated bouts of depression but also to *diabesity* — pediatric endocrinologist Dr. Francine Kaufman's term for the deadly combination of diabetes and obesity — where he easily could've landed had he not accepted Tom's unwavering urging to keep his body strong and his outlook *up.*

David is now off antidepressants because he no longer needs them, and is on his way to college. Tom seizes every opportunity to help David hold on to his physical and emotional strength. During their last visit, Tom reminded him, "Your one true power is that you can decide what you need to do in your life. Just hold that attitude, and keep making change. If you can make a small change, you can make a big change. If you can make one change, you can make another. And you build on it." Tom is gratified to watch David's own budding *sisu,* and really knew David was getting better when the young man started to challenge the doctor on meeting his own health goals. So was Dr. Allmon exercising enough? Sadly, like many physicians, no. But David's urging did spur Tom to get with the program and make some changes himself!

Wherever we are on the spectrum of health risk, we can follow the paths that Jason and his roommate, David and Dr. Allmon, and many others have shown us to maneuver our outlook, and our health, in an upward spiral.

8

COMMUNITY OUTLOOK: ALL TOGETHER NOW

Aspects of outlook can be contagious, and just as one person can serve as ground zero for the spread of a disease, a single person with a healthy attitude can have a halo effect on friends, family, neighbors, and coworkers . . . and you see where it can go from there. Practically speaking, that means that a whole family, community, or even a town and state can share in a collective outlook. Earlier, I introduced social network experts Drs. Nicholas Christakis and James Fowler, who have produced widely acclaimed research showing how aspects of our psyche, such as happiness, as well as health behaviors, such as smoking and obesity, can propagate like waves through a social network, changing the characteristics of the entire group over a period of years.

We can see the positive ripple effects of an individual on members of a group in our own social circles. In chapter 6, I gave the example of Dr. Kapoor, whose incremental optimism, built up over decades, benefited his family, friends, students, and faculty, including me. We also saw how Susan's friendliness and compassion, which had been nurtured and shaped by her own guides, inspired her to sow seeds of optimism and confidence in the minds of the most vulnerable young people in the community — people who are the future of that community. In some of those kids, these seeds will take, sprout, and grow into healthier patterns of thinking and feeling, as well as smarter behaviors, which in turn set them up for a better health span and a longer life span. When we learn to see the interconnectedness of things in this way, we understand how a positive attitude in one person can benefit countless others, because every person who is able to look *up* to mental and physical health gives herself maximal opportunity to develop her unique talents. Whenever even one of us can accomplish this feat, it not only stokes the enthusiasm of the entire group but also adds to our collective resources. To this end, cultivating a healthy outlook may perhaps be society's ultimate return on investment.

ONE PERSON'S OUTLOOK CAN
SAVE THOUSANDS OF LIVES

I saw this remarkable process in the living example of Dr. Janet Davison Rowley, who in 2011 was dubbed by the *New York Times* "the matriarch of modern cancer genetics" for her discoveries that broken chromosomes were implicated in leukemias. Thanks in part to her work, one of the most widely known of these cancers, chronic myelogenous leukemia (CML), now has a cure. But back in the early days, things weren't always so rosy for Dr. Rowley, who faced perhaps more than her fair share of ambivalence and even scorn from some of her peers. Looking back, her outlook was one of the assets that helped carry her through these scientifically trying times. During a 2012 visit to her Hyde Park home on the campus where I began my own outlook journey twenty years earlier as a student undergoing heart surgery, I spoke with Dr. Rowley about some of the fascinating personal details of her publically celebrated career.

I first met Dr. Rowley, the Blum-Riese Distinguished Service Professor of Medicine, Molecular Genetics, and Cell Biology and Human Genetics at the University of Chicago, in 1996 when she gave the commencement address at my medical school graduation. Back then she was already considered a rock star in the science world. Now in her late eighties, having been decorated by the prestigious Presidential Medal of Freedom, Lasker Award, and many other accolades, she is a living, breathing page out of the history book of cancer genetics. In the early 1970s, when I was still in cloth diapers, Dr. Rowley conducted research that revolutionized our understanding of cancer as a genetic disease, and her discoveries laid the groundwork for the world's first precisely targeted anticancer drug, imatinib (codeveloped by biochemist Nicholas Lydon and oncologist Brian Druker, with whom she shared the Japan Prize in 2012), which is now standard in the treatment of CML and several other cancers. Before imatinib, patients with CML could expect to live only a few years. Today the five-year survival rate is close to 90 percent.

Dr. Rowley became interested in chromosomes in the late 1950s when she was working part-time at a clinic in Cook County helping mentally challenged children, some of whom had Down syndrome. Back then, the concept that a chromosomal abnormality (now known as trisomy 21) could cause a clinical condition such as Down syndrome was revolutionary. In working with these children, Dr. Rowley literally saw the faces of this chromosomal abnormality, and through that human connection, she became forever hooked on understanding the genetic origins of disease. Shifting gears from her position as a part-time clinical doctor, she officially began her research career.

With the enthusiasm of "a kid in a candy store," as she aptly described herself to me, a then-fortysomething Dr. Rowley spent countless hours peering into her microscope, enraptured by the shape and appearance of chromosomes from dozens of leukemia patients. Gradually she turned her burgeoning knowledge of cytogenetics to the study of cancer, obliging her colleagues in oncology who sometimes asked her to take a look at the chromosomes of leukemia patients. In the nucleus of the cells taken from CML patients, Dr. Rowley discovered a *translocation,* or "swap," between chromosomes 9 and 22, in which little bits of the arms had broken off and traded places. This recognition in 1973 opened the door to our current understanding of CML as a genetic disease. Several decades later, with the accumulated knowledge from key scientists, we now know that this DNA swap results in a fusion oncogene (cancer-causing gene), which in turn codes for an abnormal protein leading to uncontrolled cell growth (cancer). In the five years after Dr. Rowley's initial discovery, she went on to uncover chromosomal translocations in two other leukemias. One of them, acute myelogenous leukemia (AML), is the same disease that claimed the life of my patient Ryan, from chapter 5, in 1996.

The scientific reception to Dr. Rowley's 1973 discovery of the CML translocation was lukewarm at best, with one major scientific journal even rejecting her work as "unimportant." Dr. Rowley has never been one to self-aggrandize, and on the contrary, told me "I have often been accused of being too humble," a characteristic that may have contributed to the temporary feeling of underappreciation from some of her colleagues. (Even to this day, she describes herself as "a very ordinary person with some extraordinary life circumstances.") But she remained steadfast in her conviction that the work was important, which helped keep any serious self-doubt in check.

She had several other factors on her side. First, there was her continued wonder and amazement each time she peered into her microscope. She described to me her state of mind as one of hope and excitement: "It was just sort of this optimistic enthusiasm that these findings could have an impact on the research I was doing, and on future research." She had a strong hunch that the translocations were not only associated with the leukemias, but integral to the disease process, although she was not able to prove that at the time because the DNA sequencing technology to crack the code of the fusion gene had not been developed. She was drawn to keep studying the translocations in as many types of leukemia patients as she could.

Luckily, Dr. Rowley also had the moral and material support of several close collaborators in the oncology department. She soon discovered a third translocation between chromosomes 15 and 17 in a rarer form of leukemia called acute promyelocytic leukemia (APL, a subtype of Ryan's AML). But there was a snafu, and she described herself as temporarily "heartbroken" when the pathologist informed her that the patients in whom she had identified this newest translocation had been incorrectly diagnosed and did not in fact have APL, because their cells did not have the characteristic granules — small cellular containers — necessary for that diagnosis. One of Dr. Rowley's junior colleagues at the time was

Dr. Harvey Golomb, whom I later came to know as a favorite attending (senior physician) and chairman of medicine during my residency training. Dr. Golomb remained convinced that these patients did in fact have APL, and he went the distance to get transmission electron micrographs (very high magnification) to prove it. Drs. Rowley and Golomb were now able to see the elusive, very small cytoplasmic granules of APL, thus confirming the existence of a third translocation.

Now Dr. Rowley knew she and her colleagues were on to something: "So here we had a translocation that seemed to be uniquely associated with APL, and at that point, with three findings in three types of leukemia, I decided translocations *were* important." Buoyed by the support of her colleagues, who, she told me, were not only her intellectual partners but also "treasured, treasured friends," she was imbued with vigor to keep arguing her case. She organized her research agenda around the intention (remember that concept and its role in pushing us forward toward our goal?) to document and discover what was happening at those chromosomal breakpoints. The care of leukemia as we know it today was shaped in large part by her discoveries, and thousands of people have been touched and saved by her work.

Dr. Rowley's path is an illustration of how our own outlook — and what it helps us accomplish — can influence not only our own health and aging, but the health and aging of others.

GROUP OUTLOOK: A FUTURE TOOL OF PUBLIC HEALTH

Some facets of Dr. Rowley's outlook, such as her optimism and strong sense of purpose, were readily apparent in our conversations. Other aspects took a little more consideration to categorize. A few days after interviewing Dr. Rowley in her home, I casually described her remarkable persona to personality psychologist Dr. Sarah Hampson, whom I was visiting at the Oregon Research Institute. "It's some combination of enthusiasm and doggedness," I told her. She immediately recognized the persistence as a subconstruct of trait conscientiousness. What if we could bottle some of the enthusiasm, persistence, and hopefulness — a general "I can!" — that we see in people like Dr. Rowley and so many others, and pour it into the drinking water, just like fluoride, to benefit the entire community?

As we've already seen, the life that follows

from a definitive "I can't" is not what any of us would want for our ourselves or our children. What if problem solving — and the attitudinal stance of "I can" inherently contained therein — became part of a formal curriculum to encourage both children and adults to adopt "healthier" attitudes toward their own health, and consciously set themselves on a path to healthy aging? Such an idea may seem far-fetched, but experts are already in hot pursuit of effective ways to do just that. In 2011, scientists at the National Institute on Aging (a division of the NIH), Drs. David Reiss and Lisbeth Nielsen, organized a Workshop on Conscientiousness and Healthy Aging to review the state of the science and to brainstorm methods to increase conscientiousness in children and adults, and test whether these interventions may improve health span and life span. The workshop resulted in numerous concept papers, now being published, that map out this line of research.

While the particulars of *how* one most effectively goes about instilling such character traits in children still need to be worked out, the fact that levels of conscientiousness and other traits do change over time even without our effort demonstrates that they can change, and so may be amenable to alteration with effort if we are so inclined. In a similar vein, Dr. Martin Seligman, whose widely known work I introduced briefly in chapter 1, has developed and is testing the Penn Resiliency Program in different populations. In one study, in a matter of months, school-age kids were taught to see things less pessimistically, with a measurable reduction in their future risk of mental health problems. Newer programs such as the Kindness Curriculum, developed by educator Judith Anne Rice (and described in her book of the same name) to strengthen social relationships in kids by developing greater empathy, compassion, and sharing, are currently being studied in public schools in Madison, Wisconsin. The research is led by Dr. Richard Davidson (whom I first introduced in chapter 1), director of the Center for Investigating Healthy Minds within the Waisman Center at the University of Wisconsin-Madison. Preliminary results of this project are expected in the near future.

OUTLOOK: A VISION
FOR THE ROAD AHEAD

There are fewer studies designed to deliberately change aspects of outlook to improve a physical health condition, although the landmark Recurrent Coronary Prevention Project Study did target type A behavior via special counseling involving relaxation and cognitive therapy, and subjects who underwent this treatment had a lower risk of recurrent heart attack compared with people who received standard cardiac advice. In describing outlook "management" for a population, I'm not talking about creating Stepford communities of shiny, happy people. Rather, through formal, practical instruction on attitudinally based processes like problem-solving skills and other methods we can use to regulate our negative emotions and cultivate positive ones, kids and adults alike would gain skills to manage their pessimism, hostility, or low level of conscientiousness, before it manages them. The end goal? To dream big and develop the strategies, resourcefulness, and persistence to see at least some of those dreams through. Staying as healthy as possible is a necessary part of this goal.

Cultivating the attitudes of an entire community through systematic programs may sound novel and even fringy, but conceptually, it is in keeping with standard public health approaches that have been the cornerstone of improved health span and life span in the United States for more than a century. To understand this framework more clearly, I turned to my friend, mentor, and colleague Dr. Lewis Kuller, distinguished professor of epidemiology at the University of Pittsburgh Graduate School of Public Health. Despite "retiring," Dr. Kuller continues to teach, conduct research, and mentor students and faculty alike. He is also a founding principal investigator of the Women's Health Initiative, the large dataset he and I analyzed with Dr. Karen Matthews to learn about the relative cardiovascular health and longevity of optimists, as compared to pessimists. (In fact, this project was the first in a line of research studies that inspired me to write this book.)

Teaching the Epidemiological Basis for Disease Control class he has directed for three decades, Dr. Kuller describes the science of epidemiology (the study of disease in a population) using the following medical analogy: "You could look at a community — like Pittsburgh, Allegheny County, Pennsylvania, or the United States — as your patient, much like a physician would look at any individual person, and ask the question, 'Is the patient healthy or sick? And how do you measure whether the patient is healthy or sick? If they're sick, what's wrong with them?' And so you can look at the community this way as well. I always teach that you learn the most from epidemiology by discovering differences in your community, much like a physician learns the most by studying the abnormal and comparing it to the normal." Linking this principle of comparison back to outlook, what I told you earlier about the cardiovascular health of optimists was in relation to that of pessimists, and vice versa. To be clear, neither pessimists nor optimists are abnormal, but there are marked differences in health between the two groups, and recall that we saw the largest differences between people who were farthest apart on the outlook globe.

Dr. Kuller underscores how a combined public health and traditional preventive medicine approach is needed to control cardiovascular disease and other "long incubation period" diseases that develop over decades and that are seriously threatening the health of our world population. In the case of cardiovascular disease, this long incubation period is why most people don't have heart attacks before fifty. In between birth and "the big one," there are numerous opportunities to reduce one's risk, just as we've talked about.

In public health approaches, explains Dr. Kuller, "You're not only thinking about any single individual, but every member of the population gets 'treated.' For example, to combat obesity, you build dietary change into the system — such as putting a tax on sugary drinks or prohibiting sixteen-ounce sodas from being sold — so that people make healthier choices. That's a public health effort that affects everybody, and tries to reduce obesity in the population." Dr. Kuller distinguishes this public health approach from one of preventive medicine. "A public health approach is different from a preventive medicine approach, in which a doctor counsels an individual overweight or diabetic patient to avoid the sixteen-ounce sugary drink and choose a glass of water instead." The public health approach to cultivation of outlook might involve systematic teaching of simple CBT or mindfulness principles in grade schools (similar to the Kindness Curriculum that Dr. Davidson and colleagues are studying) to help children learn to process their emotions in healthy ways and stay *up* more of the time. Individuals of all ages could supplement these public health approaches by cultivating their own attitudes through modeling parents, friends, and other exemplary individuals, by employing the 7 Steps of Attitudinal Change, by seeing a counselor, by their own preferred methods, or by a combination thereof.

Systematically rolling out outlook improvement interventions through school or community-based programs could be the ultimate "psychological immunization," as Dr. Seligman first described in the opening of his book *The Optimistic Child. Psychological immunization* is a term coined by Dr. Jonas Salk, developer of the polio vaccine, to explain the process of acquiring protective psychological traits to combat pessimism and depression. Taking this a step further and applying it more broadly to *all* aspects of outlook, the concept is as follows: Just as vaccines spur our immune systems to create antibodies against polio, pneumonia, influenza, hepatitis, and other diseases that have historically caused epidemics and even pandemics, facets of our outlook such as conscientiousness, optimism, openness, and self-compassion could arm us with the tools to cope with life's hardships.

Now take this brilliant idea one step further, and consider how "vaccinating" individuals with a healthier outlook could effectively protect them against cardiovascular disease and other chronic conditions. Take it another step further to consider that outlook vaccination may bolster the attitude latitude of the entire group, yielding what in immunological terms is called *herd immunity*. Herd immunity occurs when a critical percentage of individuals in the population — typically thought to be a threshold of around 75 percent, but possibly as low as about 45 percent — have immunity to a given disease. When this happens, even if the disease strikes, fewer and fewer individuals are susceptible, and the disease fails to gain traction in the group and fizzles out. The result? Epidemic avoided. Drs. Christakis and Fowler have shown us that social networks can serve to "transmit" aspects of our psychology and behavior from one person to the next. Drs. Hampson, Matthews, and others have in turn demonstrated that the development of cardiovascular disease risk factors and behaviors, such as smoking, obesity, and hypertension, are influenced by outlook. By managing our collective outlook in healthier ways, it is possible that as a society we would be able to effectively interrupt the cardiovascular disease process.

That doesn't necessarily mean we need 75 percent of the population to be model optimists and conscientious folk. Rather, just as with most public health interventions, a shift of just a few degrees in attitude latitude may be enough to effect a major change in cardiovascular disease rates across the nation. What will be very interesting in the future is to formally study how having a critical mass of individuals with a certain outlook — those who are looking *up* through a lens of optimism, conscientiousness, compassion, openness, etc. — may facilitate the healthy behaviors and hinder unhealthy ones to benefit the health of the whole group.

Such an undertaking may begin to sound Orwellian: What if kids became branded as "angry," "pessimistic," or "unconscientious," and then were kept down or held back as a consequence of those labels? This is certainly an important consideration, but as Dr. Hampson points out, any parent, schoolteacher, coach, or camp counselor knows that we already cultivate children's attitudes to a certain extent. "It's called upbringing," she says as we both laugh at this obvious truth. Individually, these leaders see where kids' outlooks may need guidance, and then provide it as best they can through extra help in classes at school, extra coaching on the field, assertiveness training, etc. And as Susan showed us in chapter 6, there are systems in place to identify, track, and intervene on the psychological tendencies we see in children in order to help them do better. The topic becomes more complicated when these psychological tendencies are inextricably linked to a child's socioeconomic circumstances.

OUTLOOK AND SOCIOECONOMIC STATUS (SES)

Our outlook is the product of our genes and our life experiences: Recall that I described in chapter 1 how we metabolize the world one situation at a time. Moment to moment, our outlook can be intertwined with our life circumstances, whether we're focused on a work task (we may be stressed or excited), planning for a vacation (hopeful), or doing something else. But under these surface ups and downs rest the general tendencies that make up our outlook, and these tendencies are strongly influenced by our SES — the educational, social, and especially the financial resources at our disposal. These resources, or lack thereof, are now understood to affect our health (independent of our outlook), and they do so along a gradient, with better health span and longer life span among those with the greatest resources. Much of this gradient can be explained by the clustering of traditional risk factors for cardiovascular disease and cancer with which you are now familiar. Poor and less educated people occupying less prestigious social positions, such as a lower-ranking job, tend to have more of these risk factors, while those with higher SES have fewer risk factors.

Dr. Kuller points out why this clustering of burden among lower-SES individuals is such a problem. "Epidemics," he says, "especially behavioral ones such as smoking and obesity, have their origins in better educated or higher-SES groups. Over many decades, they tend to move toward lower-SES groups, and a substantial socioeconomic gradient develops. The behavior then becomes stigmatized. Unfortunately, people of lower SES often lack the resources to successfully deal with the adverse behavior. One might even see this and mistake it as resistance to getting well, but it is in fact often associated with a lack of options."

Our outlook is linked to our SES: In the study of optimism and heart disease in almost one hundred thousand American women that I told you about in chapter 1, the most optimistic women were wealthier and more highly educated. This optimism-

SES link has been documented in people from other countries as well. Dr. Kathryn Robb and colleagues at University College London studied additional nuances of how optimism and pessimism relate to SES in a large sample of English and Scottish subjects, and found some surprising results. When the researchers examined the full LOT-R scale (which as you recall considers optimism on one end of the spectrum and pessimism on the other), and calculated the scores across four categories of SES from lowest to highest, they saw that people of greater means tended to be more optimistic than people of lesser means. In both Scotland and England, the LOT-R scores of the richest people were on average about three points higher than those of the poorest people. Recall that even a one-point difference in attitude latitude translates into measurable differences in the risk of poor health, so three points is actually a big deal healthwise.

However, when the researchers considered optimism and pessimism separately — as I have already shown you with some of my own research — they found that higher pessimism, and not lower optimism, was driving this relationship. They concluded that "lower SES people view the future in a strikingly more negative light but are almost as likely as higher SES groups to expect good events in the future." For any program to be truly effective in comprehensively helping people of lower SES, it will need to accomplish multiple daunting tasks, not the least of which is to ease some of their financial burden, which we'll discuss further. In addition, if lower SES truly drives outlook down, as it appears to do, then any intervention would need to help people either reduce their psychological negativity, increase their positivity, or both. Dr. Robb's findings for optimism and pessimism suggest that the former — decreasing pessimism — may be the more effective place to start. If poor people expect a dismal future, seeing no hope of anything better, they may be less motivated to modify their current health risk factors. (The "I have to die of something" mentality we already discussed.) Finding ways to help them dial down their high pessimism seems to be a key part of closing the health gap between rich and poor.

How might one do this? One randomized housing mobility experiment called the Moving to Opportunity Study showed that moving residents out of extreme-poverty neighborhoods (in which about half the people were poor) and into mixed-income neighborhoods (where only about one third were poor) resulted not only in lower rates of diabetes, obesity, anxiety, and stress, but also a greater sense of well-being. Researchers did not publish information on change in outlook, per se, but it begs the question of how much hopefulness (among other aspects of outlook) may have changed among those who moved up, and if so, how much such changes may have contributed to feeling *up.*

It is widely known that poor people are often subject to an accumulation of overwhelmingly stressful circumstances that can easily engender hopelessness (David Brooks's "psychology of scarcity"). In this setting, hopelessness could be reasonably viewed as a logical conclusion drawn from the surrounding data. In other words, who *wouldn't* feel hopeless with a mountain of debt, no health insurance, and no relief in sight? Dr. Karen Matthews, my colleague at the University of Pittsburgh (whose work I introduced in chapter 1), recently summarized the research on SES and health over a person's life span, citing evidence that negative personality traits, including neuroticism and hostility, are an important pathway through which the trappings of low

SES may do us biological harm. Incidentally, Dr. Matthews is the wife and colleague of Dr. Scheier, who brought us the LOT-R to measure dispositional optimism. Together and separately, through their own research as well as the training they have provided to others (including me), these two have contributed synergistically to our current understanding of the psychological and social forces at work in our bodies.

Dr. Matthews's work suggests that a low-SES environment actually engenders negative outlook traits, and she discusses these findings within the framework of the Reserve Capacity Model, which describes how low SES leads to lower *reserve capacity*. Dr. Matthews explains this concept in her own words. "I think of reserve capacity as a bank savings account that one develops to use at times of extreme stress or need," she says. "Lower-SES people may have smaller accounts, because they 'withdraw' more often due to difficult life circumstances. They also may have less to contribute to their account due to fewer educational opportunities, and perhaps less opportunity to learn life skills, including the 'skill' of being optimistic. Reserve capacity, just like in our own bank accounts, is not fixed but fluid, and changes with challenges, life stresses, and new learning." Understandably, lower reserve capacity leads to a preponderance of negative thoughts and feelings and a lower proportion of positive thoughts and feelings. This unfavorable balance fuels more fight-or-flight activation, unhealthy behaviors, and, eventually, increased disease and death.

It's no wonder University of Michigan professor Dr. Arline Geronimus referred to this sustained downward spiral and accompanying overactive stress biology as "weathering." In the same way the weather (wind, rain) erodes a mountain or a home, the ills of lower SES wear on us as well. It's important to understand that the relationships between low SES, high stress and negative outlook, and poor health are not one-way streets. Just as low SES can set the stage for fatalism, anger, depression, and other negative patterns, these same psychological tendencies may also adversely influence our SES by keeping us from fully embracing opportunities to build our resources.

THE "STATUS SYNDROME"

To further understand the links between outlook, socioeconomic status, and health, I spoke with Sir Michael Marmot, M.D., M.P.H., Ph.D., professor of epidemiology and public health at University College London and chair of the World Health Organization's Commission on Social Determinants of Health to study the root causes of inequalities in health in England and the world. Dr. Marmot led the famous Whitehall studies of British civil servants, which uncovered the inverse social gradient in disease and death, meaning that people of lower rank had higher rates of both disease and death than people of higher rank. He is also leading the English Longitudinal Study of Ageing (ELSA) and has compiled many of these research findings into his popular book, *The Status Syndrome: How Social Standing Affects our Health and Longevity,* which explains that socioeconomic status influences health to such a degree that SES is a veritable syndrome. And while lower SES portends the poorest health, we are *all* affected by the status syndrome: "At all levels of income, health and illness follow a social gradient: The lower the socioeconomic position, the worse the health."

"If it's the case that personality is thought to be genetic and unchangeable, then we're sunk," says Dr. Marmot, asserting that, luckily, aspects of the environment *do* shape our outlook and that we are not entirely at the mercy of our genes. "We need to know when and how to intervene." This is critical if we are to maximally leverage outlook as a tool to improve public health. As I alluded to earlier, research has not progressed far enough for health care providers to be able to definitively prescribe instructions for *all* aspects of outlook change and tailor these instructions to specific populations. For example, the right age at which to shape outlook is a big question on everyone's mind, including Dr. Marmot's. "I've been saying all along that early childhood is very important, but I'm not of the view that we should be throwing away everybody beyond early childhood to the scrap heap," he says, injecting a little levity into the somewhat grim reality of the socioeconomic gradient in health. "We shouldn't say, 'It's too late, we'll just wait for the next generation.' "

Sir Michael's position, articulated in 2008 and more recently in the 2012 summary of the Commission on Social Determinants of Health published in *The Lancet,* is that governments and individuals alike should work to close the health gap between individuals of low and high SES over the next generation. The commission's overarching recommendations are to: "1) improve daily living conditions, 2) tackle the inequitable distribution of power, money, and resources, and 3) measure and understand the problem and assess the results of action by establishing health-equity surveillance systems" (in other words, tracking progress as we close the SES gap). Dr. Marmot's research supports the hypothesis that aspects of our outlook help explain how SES affects our health span and life span. In addition, researchers at University of Michigan, the RAND Corporation, the Ohio State University, and other groups have demonstrated that the SES of the neighborhood we live in, over and above our own SES, influences our risk of cardiovascular disease and death. Thus, we see that there is evidence that both the care of individual people *and* the care of communities and neighborhoods are important to make a real dent in health disparities influenced by outlook and SES. The fact that psychosocial factors such as pessimism are heavily tied to our individual SES — and possibly our neighborhood SES — argues for what Dr. Marmot suggested in a poignant 2001 *New England Journal of Medicine* editorial as two logical areas of intervention to improve inequalities in health across populations: "enhancing the social and psychological resources of individual people, and improving the quality of neighborhoods and communal life."

Finally, in addition to everything we've discussed so far about outlook, SES, health, and aging, to me some of the most exciting research in this area will be to study the extent to which protective aspects of our outlook, such as optimism, may blunt some of the detrimental effects of low SES on our minds and our bodies. For example, the premature "weathering" due to low reserve capacity may not be as profound for a low-income optimist as for a low-income pessimist, especially since optimism is associated with better coping and healthier behaviors. While this question needs to be sussed out with further research, we can look to striking examples of real people who seem to answer it with a resounding yes.

THE MAN FROM UPTOWN WHO REFUSED TO BE BLINDSIDED

Consider the case of Michael Oher, the famous offensive tackle for the Baltimore Ravens whom America and the world grew to love upon learning his amazing life story through the movie *The Blind Side* and his own frank rendition, *I Beat the Odds: From Homelessness to* The Blind Side *and Beyond*. As you may know, Michael was born

341

into a world of poverty, drug addiction, imprisonment, murder, and chaos in Hurt Village, a housing project in an area of Memphis called Uptown. Placed in foster care at the age of seven, he moved from home to home, and in between various foster families weathered periods of homelessness, which likely weathered him, too. It would have been easy to let such a life crush him. Yet instead, as he tells in his autobiography, his determination and hope prevailed, catapulting him into an adulthood of material and spiritual success — what he describes as "the mind-set I had to succeed, with or without anyone's help." This inner strength allowed him to eventually revisit the horrors of his childhood — to which he had temporarily turned a blind eye for sheer emotional protection — in order to "share those memories with others so that people can learn and understand what growing up is really like for kids like me."

The American Academy of Pediatrics (AAP) has a name for Michael's childhood environment: *toxic stress.* In 2012 the AAP released a report and policy statement titled *The Lifelong Effects of Early Childhood Adversity and Toxic Stress* detailing how conditions very similar to what Michael endured barrage the body and mind. Written from the broad understanding of the human life course, the report underscores how "many adult diseases [such as cardiovascular disease and some cancers] should be viewed as developmental disorders that begin early in life and that persistent health disparities associated with poverty, discrimination, or maltreatment could be reduced by the alleviation of toxic stress in childhood."

As we've discussed, the diseases with long incubation periods begin very early, and the patterns of stress response that trigger an unhealthy physiologic environment, flooding the body with a tsunami of fight-or-flight hormones and unhealthy behaviors, serve to accelerate the disease process. Dr. Kuller emphasizes the need to balance our understanding of how psychological factors influence the development of cardiovascular disease with the understanding that they aren't the only factor: "The pessimist who doesn't smoke, takes medicine to control blood pressure and lipids, and follows a healthy diet will do better than the optimist who smokes and drinks at the bar eating pickled pig's feet, without a care to his hypertension and cholesterol." This point is key, and it brings us back to my original premise, which is that aspects of our outlook, which tend to be shaped very early in life, precede and predict the development of the very risk factors that lead to the diseases that are most likely to result in our demise. In other words, optimists are less likely than pessimists to be sitting at the bar smoking and eating delicacies with a saturated fat content high enough to take out one of their coronary arteries.

For many children born into difficult circumstances of any kind, toxic stress strikes when the developing brain and other organs are at their most vulnerable. Our outlook may be one layer of defense that prevents toxic stress from getting too deep under our skin, buoying us until greater help in the form of friends, guides, and the SES improvements, which Dr. Marmot champions, arrives. Having emerged from this toxic stress to come full circle, Michael Oher knows firsthand the power of hope and determination, which he readily offers to the half-million kids currently in the U.S. foster care system, through charitable donations and the honesty and introspection that have made his personal story required reading in my home. He emphasizes that dreams, however small, are just as important to a kid in foster care as the big dream of Martin Luther King: "Having some kind of a goal is absolutely essential for kids trapped in poverty and bad family situations, because if we can't hope that things might be better someday, then we basically lose a reason to live." Dante wasn't kidding when he revealed to us in his epic poem *The Inferno* the command inscribed on the gate of Hell: "Abandon hope, all ye who enter here." It's not only the conditions of suffering that make our experiences more hellish — they become so when there is no hope of anything else. Which is what makes individuals like Michael, who staunchly refused to follow that inscription, so fascinating and inspiring.

LOOKING FORWARD

For now, there are no standardized guidelines for clinicians or public health officials
to follow as they promote attitudinal change.
In the absence of such guidelines, anyone
wanting to move attitude latitude can utilize
the strategies I've laid out here and accept
my invitation to develop your own strategies
to reach these goals. In the future, I hope to
conduct clinical trials to produce the data
needed for clinical guidelines, and to actually help write them. Until that happens, it
is unethical in my eyes to leave people hanging, especially when it is virtually inconceiv-
able that anyone would be harmed by
adopting a motivated, engaged, and more
hopeful (or less unhopeful) outlook that
propels them toward healthy aging. While
clinical trials are underway, people of all
ages should be encouraged to cultivate their
outlook in healthy ways. As Dr. George Vail-
lant has shown us through the nine-decade

Harvard Grant Study he directs, we truly can "triumph" at any age, regardless of what our lives were like as younger people.

You've already taken the first step in your outlook journey by reading this book and in doing so, opening yourself up to new ways of thinking and feeling. Maybe you've even already moved to healthier ground. Remember that this may take time: Not everyone automatically wakes up in the morning with their outlook button set to "full speed ahead." After taking great pains to become consciously aware of our outlook so that we can change it for the better, the ultimate goal is to make this new and improved lens on the world an unconscious habit. In the meantime, think of your outlook as a newly discovered muscle that may turn out to be the most powerful one in your body — and certainly one that you can tone and strengthen — by starting out slowly, and working your way *up.*

ACKNOWLEDGMENTS

Those who espouse the Buddhist principle of interconnectedness, as I do, know that this book comprises elements from all my life experiences that, collectively, have made me who I am today, and that have found their way onto these pages through my fingers. I do not even consciously remember some of the people, animals, and places that have gotten me to this point, yet I can still acknowledge the role they have played. The late Dr. Karl Weintraub, one of my most beloved teachers, instilled in me a deep appreciation for the value of the individual, but at the same he taught me how individuals are a product of the civilizations in which they have been brought up. So my first nod is to every thread of this broader context, and especially to my parents, Phyllis Janik and Harold Tinkle, who for me made up the bulk of it. I try to follow their courageous example of composing my thoughts

349

on the page, like Tagore's bird of faith, singing "while the dawn is still dark."

I am certain my heart would have stopped
pumping somewhere around age twenty-
five were it not for the efforts of the cardiology, anesthesiology, and cardiovascular
surgery teams who cared for me at the
University of Chicago, including Dr. Victoria Nevins, who first auscultated my
murmur; Dr. Roberto Lang, who circulated
copies of my echocardiogram internation-
ally to develop a treatment plan for my rare
condition; Dr. Duane Follman, who performed my cardiac catheterization; Dr.
Long Han, who oversaw my blood pressure
and respirations on bypass; and, of course,
the late Dr. Robert Karp and his then-
partner, Dr. Greg Sand, along with their
then-trainee, Dr. Mario Albertucci. A special thanks to Dr. Karp for wearing the head
camera that provided me with a priceless
visual record of this defining life event.

The help I received along the protracted
journey of book writing has made it that
much easier to walk the path. I tip my hat
first to my agent, Rebecca Gradinger, who
also introduced me to Tula Karras, my
independent editor. Rebecca landed this
work on the desk of Caroline Sutton and
later Christina Rodriguez, my editors at

Hudson Street Press. Rebecca and Caroline, particular thanks go to you both for taking a chance on this unproven horse! The editorial efforts, which began with Rebecca's tireless suggestions on earlier versions and culminated with Tula's and Christina's magic shears and the expert edits from my mom, have shaped the writing far beyond where I could have taken it alone. Without the support of these women, the work simply would not have materialized. I also wish to thank Jaya Miceli from the art department for the cover design, Brittney Ross and Meghan Stevenson for their editorial assistance, and all members of the production crew — including John Fagan and Ashley Pattison in marketing, Liz Keenan and Courtney Nobile in publicity, and Kym Surridge, who performed meticulous and thoughtful copyediting — for the gargantuan efforts in churning out the final product.

In addition to many colleagues whom I already acknowledged in the book proper, I am indebted to the academic mentors, colleagues, and health care providers at different institutions who have taught me, especially Mr. Tony Paris, Ms. Linda Kennedy, Mr. Greg Harris, Dr. Edward Wingler, Dr. Herbert Friedman and the Drs. Strauss for their exquisite biology training during my undergraduate years; Dr. Arthur Rubenstein, who has helped guide my career over two decades through many windy paths; Dr. Holly Humphrey, whose tutelage and residency training program shaped me into the clinician I am today; Dr. Jesse Hall, who was the first to encourage me to train in medicine, and who also predicted my writing career when I was yet a student; Drs. David Eisenberg and Russell Phillips for their guidance during fellowship training; Dr. Sara Lazar, Dr. Julie Fiez, Dr. Dick Jennings, and especially Dr. Saul Shiffman, my primary mentor in tobacco research, who has guided a great deal of my work over the last eight years at the University of Pittsburgh. I would also like to thank Dr. Steve Reis, Director of the Clinical and Translational Science Institute (CTSI), who validated a series of "thirty-degree turns" along my research path. The CTSI itself has supported my research over the past eight years. Following the call of the NIH to *translate* published evidence into practice, I view this book as a *tool of translation,* and one that I hope will encourage many people to put the science into action for the benefit of their own health.

As for my patients — past, present, and

future — thank you for everything you've taught me. Were it not for the intense challenges of patient care, this book would never have had a reason to materialize. While my views don't necessarily represent the views of the funding agencies that have supported my research (and much of the research I've discussed within), I wish to acknowledge their pivotal role in my career: the National Institutes of Health (particularly the National Cancer Institute, the National Heart Lung and Blood Institute, the National Institute on Drug Abuse, and the National Center for Complementary and Alternative Medicine); the Mind and Life Institute, which supported me in the earliest days of my research career and provided me with the most unique mentorship incorporating both neuroscientific and Buddhist principles; the Pittsburgh Foundation Charles and Nancy Emmerling Fund; the Pittsburgh Mind Body Center; the American Legacy Foundation; and the Association of Schools of Public Health.

I am indebted to the many family members on both sides who passed countless hours with me growing up, both in Chicago and during summers in California, and especially to my grandparents Phil and Therese Janik, who picked me up from

Monroe school and made me French toast and pot roast every week; and to my great-aunt Dorothy, who has seen the earth circumnavigate the sun ninety-two times, and who still makes me feel like a teenager, worry lines and all.

My closest friends have provided a much-needed guide rope stretching across the years, including Dr. Jaime Kean, Beverly Burke, Dr. Belinda Marcus, Drs. Laurent Tao, Ralph Verdino, Vasan Ramachandran, and John A. Benson Jr., Laura Johansen, Bill and Tre Siebert, Chris and Colleen Strand, John and Connie Champion, Bob Strecker, Anita Wolff, Dr. Kristin Humphreys, Dr. Anne McCaffrey, Drs. Smita Nayak and Michael Grabe, Dr. Bruce Lee, Drs. Esa Davis and Darrell Rubin, Drs. Sam Youssem and Penny Williams, Molly Donohue and Dr. Anthony Spinola, Drs. Mark Gladwin and Tammy Shields, Drs. Martha Gulati, Savitri Fedson, Mary Rinella, Fiona Gibbons, and Nancy Torres-Finnerty, Hannah and Martin de San Martin, Andy Tran, and Kiki and Bill McConnell. To Klaus Boettcher, my own counselor, you pulled me *up* more than once! My gratitude also extends to classmates, colleagues, friends, and family who fostered my literary spirit with regular "doses" of nonmedical books and articles to remind me of life outside of the classroom, library, or hospital: Mary Ellen Janik, George and Karen Freiberg, Paul Forrester, Rick Nunziati, Dr. Michael Fretzin, Drs. Vanessa Torbensen, Imelda Dacones, Elmer Abbo, Isabel Navarrete Polsky and Charles Polsky, Dr. John McConville, Dr. Aaron Angel, Deb Seltzer, Bernard Switala, Dr. Michael Yonas, and, of course, my mother.

To Stacey Dillon, Adelina Malito, Sharon Maddox, and Lin Hough, thank you for providing comments on portions of earlier drafts of the book. To Thomas Ylioja, thanks for a complete overview.

To Matt — I'll say only that this would not have happened without you. And to my girls, Mom is finally back!

RESOURCES

You've just read over two hundred pages, so I'll keep this short. Below are a few additional resources you may find useful. It is by no means an exhaustive list. Wherever possible, I've included resources that are free or nominally-priced. Some may also be available for check-out at your local library.

Mindfulness and Self Compassion

Dr. Kristin Neff has an excellent Web site with more information on self-compassion: www.self-compassion.org

Dr. Chris Germer has free mindfulness downloads at his Web site: www.mindfulselfcompassion.org

The University of Massachusetts Center for Mindfulness is also an excellent resource for training programs, books, audio learning, ongoing research, and other mindfulness-related information: www.umassmed.eduContent.aspx?id=

42434

My friend, colleague, and veteran mindfulness instructor Micki Fine has a Web site you may enjoy: www.living mindfully.org. Micki has a forthcoming book that discusses a unique application of mindfulness, and which may be helpful for women (like me) who tend to bend a little too far backward to please others: *The Need to Please: Mindfulness Skills for Finding Freedom from People-Pleasing and Approval-Seeking* (September 2013).

Check out the Mind and Life Institute, a truly unique organization fostering scientific and practical dialogue between Buddhist leaders (including the Dalai Lama) and leading neuroscientists from around the world. www.mindandlife.org

Guided Imagery

Martin Rossman, M.D., has a Web site featuring books and audio learning for sale: www.thehealingmind.org/index

Belleruth Naparstek also has a Web site featuring her blog, audio learning, and ongoing imagery-related research: www.belleruthnaparstek.com

Contemplation

Richard Rohr has a number of books and recorded teachings available through the Center for Action and Contemplation in Albuquerque, New Mexico: www.cac.org. The bookstore, Mustard Seed, is also accessible online: www.cac.org/store. This site has many nominally priced items, including the audio teachings (with Father Keating) of contemplative prayer, and emotional sobriety, which I mentioned in chapter 4.

One More Piece of "Typical Doctor Advice"

You may enjoy this book by my colleague, friend, and cardiologist Martha Gulati (and coauthor Sherry Torkos) entitled, *Saving Women's Hearts: How You Can Prevent and Reverse Heart Disease with Natural and Conventional Strategies*. Martha's landmark research on the importance of fitness in women has earned her many national appearances.

Other

Finally, if you were as moved as I was by Jordan, the Maori man in chapter 4 who was courageous enough to face his fear of "the big picture," listen to him with your own ears on the following BBC podcast: www.bbc.co.uk/program mes/p00y8vf1 (9/29 BBC World Service; first broadcast 9/27/2012; generally available for over one year from the time of first broadcast).

NOTES

Chapter 1: How Our Outlook Drives Our Health and Aging

from how quickly we recover from an illness or surgery: H. Tindle, B. H. Belnap, P. R. Houck, et al., "Optimism, Response to Treatment of Depression, and Rehospitalization After Coronary Artery Bypass Graft Surgery," *Psychosomatic Medicine* 74, no. 2 (2012): 200–207; see also: M. F. Scheier, K. A. Matthews, J. F. Owens, et al., "Optimism and Rehospitalization After Coronary Artery Bypass Graft Surgery," *Archives of Internal Medicine* 159, no. 8 (1999): 829–35.

to whether we become depressed: E. J. Giltay, F. G. Zitman, and D. Kromhout, "Dispositional Optimism and the Risk of Depressive Symptoms During 15 Years of Follow-up: The Zutphen Elderly Study," *Journal of Affective Disorders* 91, no. 1

(2006): 45–52; see also: G. C. Patton, M. M. Tollit, H. Romaniuk, et al., "A Prospective Study of the Effects of Optimism on Adolescent Health Risks," *Pediatrics* 127, no. 2 (2011): 308–16.

develop cardiovascular risk factors: E. J. Giltay, F. G. Zitman, and D. Kromhout, "Dispositional Optimism and the Risk of Depressive Symptoms During 15 Years of Follow-up: The Zutphen Elderly Study"; see also: I. C. Siegler, B. L. Peterson, J. C. Barefoot, and R. B. Williams, "Hostility During Late Adolescence Predicts Coronary Risk Factors at Mid-life," *American Journal of Epidemiology* 136, no. 2 (1992): 146–54; and H. Nabi, M. Kivimaki, S. Sabia, et al., "Hostility and Trajectories of Body Mass Index Over 19 Years: The Whitehall II Study," *American Journal of Epidemiology* 169, no. 3 (2008): 347–54.

or suffer a heart attack: J. D. Newman, K. W. Davidson, J. A. Shaffer, et al., "Observed Hostility and the Risk of Incident Ischemic Heart Disease," *JACC: Journal of the American College of Cardiology* 58, no. 12 (2011): 1222–28; see also H. A. Tindle, Y. F. Chang, L. H. Kuller, et al., "Optimism, Cynical Hostility, and Incident Coronary Heart Disease and Mortality in the Women's Health Initia-

tive," *Circulation* 120, no. 8 (2009): 656–
62; and Y. Chida and A. Steptoe, "The Association of Anger and Hostility with Future Coronary Heart Disease: A Meta-analytic Review of Prospective Evidence," *JACC: Journal of the American College of Cardiology* 53, no. 11 (2009): 936–46.

stroke: H. Nabi, M. Koskenvuo, A. Singh-Manoux, et al., "Low Pessimism Protects Against Stroke: The Health and Social Support (HeSSup) Prospective Cohort Study," *Stroke* 41, no. 1 (2010): 187–90.

or cancer: Y. Chida, M. Hamer, J. Wardle, and A. Steptoe, "Do Stress-Related Psychosocial Factors Contribute to Cancer Incidence and Survival?" *Nature Clinical Practice Oncology* 5, no. 8 (2008): 466–75.

when our health begins to break down: H. Tindle, et al. "Psychological Attitudes and Risk of CHD and Mortality Across Varying Levels of Risk Factor Burden," *Psychosomatic Medicine* 72 (2010): A-39; and C. S. Carver, C. Pozo-Kaderman, S. D. Harris, et al., "Optimism Versus Pessimism Predicts the Quality of Women's Adjustment to Early Stage Breast Cancer," *Cancer* 73, no. 4 (1994): 1213–20.

general expectation of good things to come: M. F. Scheier, C. S. Carver, and

M. W. Bridges, "Distinguishing Optimism from Neuroticism (and Trait Anxiety, Self-Mastery, and Self-Esteem): A Reevaluation of the Life Orientation Test," *Journal of Personality and Social Psychology* 67, no. 6 (1994): 1063–78.

published in the journal *Circulation*: Tindle, et al., "Optimism, Cynical Hostility, and Incident Coronary Heart Disease and Mortality in the Women's Health Initiative."

most people are selfish, dishonest, and unworthy: W. W. Cook and D. M. Medley, "Proposed Hostility and Pharisaic-Virtue Scales for the MMPI," *Journal of Applied Psychology* 38, no. 6 (1954): 414–18.

and does a healthy outlook actually keep us physiologically younger?: H. Tindle, E. Davis, and L. Kuller, "Attitudes and Cardiovascular Disease," *Maturitas* 67, no. 2 (2010): 108–13.

***compression of morbidity*:** J. F. Fries, "Aging, Natural Death, and the Compression of Morbidity," *New England Journal of Medicine* 303, no. 3 (1980): 245–50.

breakthroughs are happening every day: L. B. Gordon, M. E. Kleinman, D. T. Miller, et al., "Clinical Trial of a Farnesyltransferase Inhibitor in Children with

Hutchinson-Gilford Progeria Syndrome," *PNAS: Proceedings of the National Academy of Sciences,* early edition (2012):1–6.

from early childhood over their lifetime: H. S. Friedman and L. R. Martin, *The Longevity Project: Surprising Discoveries for Health and Long Life from the Landmark Eight-Decade Study* (New York: Hudson Street Press, 2011).

similar results from other populations: M. L. Kern and H. S. Friedman, "Do Conscientious Individuals Live Longer?: A Quantitative Review," *Health Psychology* 27, no. 5 (2008): 505–12; see also: A. Terracciano, C. E. Lockenhoff, A. B. Zonderman, et al., "Personality Predictors of Longevity: Activity, Emotional Stability, and Conscientiousness," *Psychosomatic Medicine* 70, no. 6 (2008): 621–27.

harbinger of risk for future heart attack: C. Iribarren, S. Sidney, D. E. Bild, et al., "Association of Hostility with Coronary Artery Calcification in Young Adults: The CARDIA Study," *JAMA: Journal of the American Medical Association* 283, no. 19 (2000): 2546–51.

develop high blood pressure in the first place: L. L. Yan, K. Liu, K. A. Matthews, M. L. Daviglus, T. F. Ferguson, and C. L. Kiefe, "Psychosocial Factors and Risk of

Hypertension: The Coronary Artery Risk Development in Young Adults (CARDIA) Study," *JAMA: Journal of the American Medical Association* 290, no. 16 (2003): 2138–48.

less neurotic counterparts to suffer dementia: P. R. Duberstein, B. P. Chapman, H. A. Tindle, et al., "Personality and Risk for Alzheimer's Disease in Adults 72 Years of Age and Older: A 6-Year Follow-up," *Psychology and Aging* 26, no. 2 (2011): 351–62; see also: B. Chapman, P. Duberstein, H. A. Tindle, et al., "Personality Predicts Cognitive Function over 7 Years in Older Persons," *American Journal of Geriatric Psychiatry* 20, no. 7 (2012): 612–21.

less likely than pessimists to suffer a stroke: Nabi, et al., "Low Pessimism Protects Against Stroke"; see also: E. S. Kim, N. Park, and C. Peterson, "Dispositional Optimism Protects Older Adults from Stroke," *Stroke* 42, no. 10 (2011): 2855–9.

more likely to recur and cause death: Chida, et al., "Do Stress-Related Psychosocial Factors Contribute?"

less likely than pessimists to become depressed: Giltay, et al., "Dispositional Optimism and the Risk of Depressive

Symptoms"; see also: G. C. Patton, M. M. Tollit, H. Romaniuk, S. H. Spence, J. Sheffield, and M. G. Sawyer, "A Prospective Study of the Effects of Optimism on Adolescent Health Risks," *Pediatrics* 127, no 2 (2011): 308–16.

Teenagers with an optimistic explanatory style: C. Peterson and M. E. Seligman, "Explanatory Style and Illness," *Journal of Personality* 55, no. 2 (1987): 237–65.

being suspended from school: Ibid.

more likely to start smoking in middle school: J. W. Weiss, M. Mouttapa, C. Chou, et al., "Hostility, Depressive Symptoms, and Smoking in Early Adolescence," *Journal of Adolescence* 28, no. 1 (2005): 49–62; see also: J. W. Weiss, M. Mouttapa, S. Cen, C. A. Johnson, and J. Unger, "Longitudinal Effects of Hostility, Depression, and Bullying on Adolescent Smoking Initiation," *Journal of Adolescent Health* 48, no. 6 (2011): 591–96.

better eating habits, and higher educational attainment: S. E. Hampson, L. R. Goldberg, T. M. Vogt, and J. P. Dubanoski, "Mechanisms by which Childhood Personality Traits Influence Adult Health Status: Educational Attainment and Healthy Behaviors," *Health Psychology* 26, no. 1 (2007): 121–25.

highest among people who have the shortest telomeres: P. Willeit, J. Willeit, A. Mayr, et al., "Telomere Length and Risk of Incident Cancer and Cancer Mortality," *JAMA: Journal of the American Medical Association* 304, no. 1 (2010): 69–75.

pessimistic people have shorter telomeres: B. Roy, A. V. Diez-Roux, T. Seeman, N. Ranjit, S. Shea, and M. Cushman, "Association of Optimism and Pessimism with Inflammation and Hemostasis in the Multi-Ethnic Study of Atherosclerosis (MESA)," *Psychosomatic Medicine* 72, no. 2 (2009): 134–40; see also: A. O'Donovan, J. Lin, F. S. J. Tillie, et al., "Pessimism Correlates with Leukocyte Telomere Shortness and Elevated Interleukin-6 in Post-Menopausal Women," *Brain, Behavior, and Immunity* 23, no. 4 (2009): 446–49.

inflammation and aging: *inflammaging:* C. Franceschi, M. Bonafe, S. Valensin, et al., "Inflamm-aging: An Evolutionary Perspective on Immunosenescence," *Annals of the New York Academy of Sciences* 908 (2000): 244–54; see also: C. Franceschi, M. Capri, D. Monti, et al., "Inflammaging and Anti-Inflammaging: A Systemic Perspective on Ageing and Longevity Emerged from Studies in Humans," *Mechanisms of Ageing and Development* 128, no. 1 (2007): 92–105.

pessimism is associated with greater inflammation: A. Ikeda, J. Schwartz, J. L. Peters, et al., "Optimism in Relation to Inflammation and Endothelial Dysfunction in Older Men: The VA Normative Aging Study," *Psychosomatic Medicine* 73, no. 8 (2011): 664–71; see also: O'Donovan, et al., "Pessimism Correlates with Leukocyte Telomere Shortness and Elevated Interleukin-6 in Post-Menopausal Women."

became stooped, slow, and weak: D. J. Baker, T. Wijshake, T. Tchkonia, et al., "Clearance of p16Ink4a-Positive Senescent Cells Delays Ageing-Associated Disorders," *Nature* 479, no. 7372 (2011): 232–36.

Molecules of Emotion: Why You Feel the Way You Feel: C. B. Pert, *Molecules of Emotion: Why You Feel the Way You Feel* (New York: Touchstone, 1997).

The End of Stress as We Know It: B. S. McEwen and E. N. Lasley, *The End of Stress as We Know It* (Washington, D.C.: National Academies Press, 2002).

The Hostage Brain: B. S. McEwen and H. M. Schmeck, Jr., *The Hostage Brain* (New York: Rockefeller University Press, 1994).

promote survival by readying us for action: B. S. McEwen, "Protective and Damaging Effects of Stress Mediators," *New England Journal of Medicine* 338, no. 3 (1998): 171–79.

the brunt of the mind's ire during fight-or-flight arousal: J. A. Arrighi, M. Burg, I. S. Cohen, et al., "Myocardial Blood-Flow Response During Mental Stress in Patients with Coronary Artery Disease," *Lancet* 356, no. 9226 (2000): 310–11; see also: M. M. Burg, B. Graeber, A. Vashist, et al., "Noninvasive Detection of Risk for Emotion-Provoked Myocardial Ischemia," *Psychosomatic Medicine* 71, no. 1 (2009): 14–20; R. Lampert, V. Shusterman, M. Burg, et al., "Anger-Induced T-Wave Alternans Predicts Future Ventricular Arrhythmias in Patients with Implantable Cardioverter-Defibrillators," *Journal of the American College of Cardiology* 53, no. 9 (2009): 774–78; R. Soufer, J. D. Bremner, J. A. Arrighi, et al., "Cerebral Cortical Hyperactivation in Response to Mental Stress in Patients with Coronary Artery Disease," *Proceedings of the National Academy of Sci-*

ences of the United States of America 95, no. 11 (1998): 6454–59; R. Soufer, H. Jain, and A. J. Yoon, "Heart-Brain Interactions in Mental Stress-Induced Myocardial Ischemia," *Current Cardiology Reports* 11, no. 2 (2009): 133–40; I. S. Wittstein, D. R. Thiemann, J. A. Lima, et al., "Neurohumoral Features of Myocardial Stunning Due to Sudden Emotional Stress," *New England Journal of Medicine* 352, no. 6 (2005): 539–48; and R. C. Ziegelstein, "Acute Emotional Stress and Cardiac Arrhythmias," *JAMA: Journal of the American Medical Association* 298, no. 3 (2007): 324–29.

dietary plan that had been recommended for them: L. F. Tinker, M. C. Rosal, A. F. Young, et al., "Predictors of Dietary Change and Maintenance in the Women's Health Initiative Dietary Modification Trial," *Journal of the American Dietetic Association* 107, no. 7 (2007): 1155–65.

the concept of "ideal cardiac health": D. M. Lloyd-Jones, Y. Hong, D. Labarthe, et al., "Defining and Setting National Goals for Cardiovascular Health Promotion and Disease Reduction: The American Heart Association's Strategic Impact Goal Through 2020 and Beyond," *Circula-*

371

tion 121, no. 4 (2010): 586–613.

50 percent chance of having a heart attack or stroke: A. R. Folsom, H. Yatsuya, J. A. Nettleton, et al., "Community Prevalence of Ideal Cardiovascular Health, by the American Heart Association Definition, and Relationship with Cardiovascular Disease Incidence," *Journal of the American College of Cardiology* 57, no. 16 (2011): 1690–96.

less than 1 percent of American adults: Ibid; see also: C. Bambs, K. F. Kip, A. Dinga, S. R. Mulukutla, A. N. Aiyer, and S. E. Reis, "Low Prevalence of 'Ideal Cardiovascular Health' in a Community-Based Population: The Heart Strategies Concentrating on Risk Evaluation (Heart SCORE) Study," *Circulation* 123, no 8 (2011): 850–57.

had better cardiovascular risk profiles than pessimists: Tindle, et al., "Optimism, Cynical Hostility, Incident Coronary Heart Disease and Mortality in the Women's Health Initiative."

to gain more weight as time went by: Nabi, et al, "Hostility and Trajectories of Body Mass Index over 19 Years: The Whitehall II Study."

one-half of our outlook can be considered genetic: R. Plomin, M. F. Scheier,

C. S. Bergeman, N. L. Pedersen, J. R. Nesselroade, and G. E. McClearn, "Optimism, Pessimism and Mental Health: A Twin/Adoption Analysis," *Personality and Individual Differences* 13, no. 8 (1992): 921–30.

character traits that comprise our outlook: R. R. McCrae and P. T. Costa, "Personality Trait Structure as a Human Universal," *American Psychologist* 52, no. 5 (1997): 509–16.

healthy ways after a disabling event: C. J. Boyce and A. M. Wood, "Personality Prior to Disability Determines Adaptation: Agreeable Individuals Recover Lost Life Satisfaction Faster and More Completely," *Psychological Science* 22, no. 11 (2011): 1397–1402.

and to exhibit antisocial behavior: S. E. Jones, J. D. Miller, D. R. Lynam, "Personality, Antisocial Behavior, and Aggression: A Meta-Analytic Review," *Journal of Criminal Justice* 39, no. 4 (2011): 329–37.

all other things being equal: T. Sone, N. Nakaya, K. Ohmori, et al., "Sense of Life Worth Living (Ikigai) and Mortality in Japan: Ohsaki Study," *Psychosomatic Medicine* 70, no. 6 (2008): 709–15.

The Emotional Life of Your Brain: How Its Unique Patterns Affect the Way You

***Think, Feel, and Live — and How You
Can Change Them:*** R. J. Davidson and S.
Begley, *The Emotional Life of Your Brain:
How Its Unique Patterns Affect the Way You
Think, Feel, and Live — and How You Can
Change Them* (New York: Hudson Street
Press, 2012).

the Holy Grail: R. Farzaneh-Far, J. Lin, E.
S. Epel, W. S. Harris, E. H. Blackburn,
and M. A. Whooley, "Association of Ma-
rine Omega-3 Fatty Acid Levels with Te-
lomeric Aging in Patients with Coronary
Heart Disease," *JAMA: Journal of the
American Medical Association* 303, no. 3
(2010): 250–57.

**purpose in life, *and* increased telom-
erase activity:** E. Epel, J. Daubenmier, J.
T. Moskowitz, S. Folkman, and E. Blackburn, "Can Meditation Slow Rate of Cellular Aging? Cognitive Stress, Mindfulness, and Telomeres," *Annals of the New
York Academy of Sciences* 1172 (2009):
34–53; see also: T. L. Jacobs, E. S. Epel, J.
Lin, et al., "Intensive Meditation Training, Immune Cell Telomerase Activity, and
Psychological Mediators," *Psychoneuroen-
docrinology* 36, no. 5 (2011): 664–81.

**the way we process our anxieties and
fears:** P. R. Porto, L. Oliveira, J. Mari, E.

Volchan, I. Figueira, and P. Ventura, "Does Cognitive Behavioral Therapy Change the Brain? A Systematic Review of Neuroimaging in Anxiety Disorders," *Journal of Neuropsychiatry and Clinical Neurosciences* 21, no. 2 (2009): 114–25; and K. Goldapple, Z. Segal, C. Garson, et al., "Modulation of Cortical-Limbic Pathways in Major Depression: Treatment-Specific Effects of Cognitive Behavior Therapy," *Archives of General Psychiatry* 61, no. 1 (2004): 34–41.

would not live beyond age thirty-five: I. W. Borowsky, M. Ireland, and M. D. Resnick, "Health Status and Behavioral Outcomes for Youth Who Anticipate a High Likelihood of Early Death," *Pediatrics* 124, no. 1 (2009): e81–e88.

positive social bonds with adults: N. N. Duke, C. L. Skay, S. L. Pettingell, and I. W. Borowsky, "Early Death Perception in Adolescence: Identifying Factors Associated with Change from Pessimism to Optimism About Life Expectancy," *Clinical Pediatrics* 50, no. 1 (2011): 21–28.

coined the term *psychological immunization*: M. E. P. Seligman, K. Reivich, L. Jaycox, and J. Gillham, *The Optimistic Child: A Proven Program to Safeguard*

Children Against Depression and Build Lifelong Resilience (Boston: Houghton Mifflin, 2007).

Chapter 2: The Many Faces of Optimism

meaning that they are essentially unrelated: N. M. Radcliffe and W. M. P. Klein, "Dispositional, Unrealistic, and Comparative Optimism: Differential Relations with the Knowledge and Processing of Risk Information and Beliefs about Personal Risk," *Personality and Social Psychology Bulletin* 28, no. 6 (2002): 836–46.

data on the lifetime risks of cardiovascular disease: J. D. Berry, A. Dyer, X. Cai, et al., "Lifetime Risks of Cardiovascular Disease," *New England Journal of Medicine* 366, no. 4 (2012): 321–29.

reduction in risk of cardiovascular disease: J. G. Robinson, C. Rahilly-Tierney, E. Lawler, and J. M. Gaziano, "Benefits Associated with Achieving Optimal Risk Factor Levels for the Primary Prevention of Cardiovascular Disease in Older Men," *Journal of Clinical Lipidology* 6, no. 1 (2012): 58–65.

first question on the Life Orientation Test, Revised (LOT-R): Scheier, et al., "Distinguishing Optimism from Neuroticism (and Trait Anxiety, Self-Mastery, and Self-Esteem): A Reevaluation of the Life Orientation Test."

recently replicated that finding in a second study: Tindle, et al., "Optimism, Response to Treatment of Depression, and Rehospitalization After Coronary Artery Bypass Graft Surgery."

Department of Health and Human Services guidelines on treating tobacco use: Tobacco Use and Dependence Guideline Panel, *Treating Tobacco Use and Dependence: 2008 Update* (Rockville, MD: U.S. Department of Health and Human Services, 2008).

"Scarcity creates its own psychology": D. Brooks, "The Unexamined Society," *New York Times,* July 7, 2011.

can affect rich and poor people alike: A. K. Shah, S. Mullainathan, and E. Shafir, "Some Consequences of Having Too Little," *Science* 338 (2012): 682–85.

Breaking Murphy's Law: How Optimists Get What They Want from Life — and Pessimists Can Too: S. C. Segerstrom, *Breaking Murphy's Law: How Optimists Get What They Want from Life — and Pessimists Can Too* (New York: The Guilford Press, 2006).

why optimists tend to adjust better:

S. C. Segerstrom, "Optimism and Attentional Bias for Negative and Positive Stimuli," *Personality and Social Psychology Bulletin* 27, no. 10: 1334–43.

endorse *ikigai* live longer than those who do not: T. Sone, et al., "Sense of Life Worth Living."

***The Optimism Bias: A Tour of the Irrationally Positive Brain*:** T. Sharot, *The Optimism Bias: A Tour of the Irrationally Positive Brain* (New York: Vintage, 2011).

a major brain network responsible for thinking and feeling: T. Sharot, A. M. Riccardi, C. M. Raio, and E. A. Phelps, "Neural Mechanisms Mediating Optimism Bias," *Nature* 450, no. 7166 (2007): 102–5.

In one of her letters in 1953: Mother Teresa, *Mother Teresa: Come Be My Light — The Private Writings of the Saint of Calcutta* (New York: Doubleday, 2007).

Chapter 3: The Savvy Outlook Traveler 1

***Self-Compassion: Stop Beating Yourself Up and Leave Insecurity Behind*:** K. Neff, *Self-Compassion: Stop Beating Yourself Up and Leave Insecurity Behind* (New York: William Morrow, 2011).

Taking the Leap: Freeing Ourselves from Old Habits and Fears: P. Chödrön, *Taking the Leap: Freeing Ourselves from Old Habits and Fears* (Boston: Shambhala, 2009).

joy is beneficial for physical health: S. D. Pressman and S. Cohen, "Positive Affect and Health," *Current Directions in Psychological Science* 15, no. 3: 122–25. J. K. Buehm and L. D. Kubzansky, "The Heart's Content: The Association Between Positive Psychological Well-Being and Cardiovascular Health." *Psychological Bulletin* 138(4), July 2012: 655–91.

brain activity *in response to* the heat probe: R. C. deCharms, "Applications of Real-Time fMRI," *Nature Reviews Neuroscience* 9 (2008): 720–29.

Chapter 4: The Savvy Outlook Traveler 2

I have adapted two of them (guided imagery and mindfulness): *Mindfulness-Based Addiction Treatment (MBAT) Manual* (2008).

New Zealand's most notorious and violent gangs: R. Kesby, BBC World Service, Auckland, "New Zealand Gangs: The Mongrel Mob and Other Urban Outlaws," link available at: http://www

.bbc.co.uk/news/magazine-19153425, September 25, 2012.

developed by American psychiatrist Dr. Aaron Beck: "Cognitive Therapy of Depression: New Perspectives," in P. Clayton, ed., *Treatment of Depression: Old Controversies and New Approaches* (New York: Raven Press, 1983), pp. 265–90; see also: A. T. Beck, *Cognitive Therapy and the Emotional Disorders* (New York: International Universities Press, 1976).

without actively trying to change them: J. Kabat-Zinn, *Full Catastrophe Living: Using the Wisdom of Your Body and Mind to Face Stress, Pain, and Illness* (New York: Dell, 1990).

***Mindfulness Based Cognitive Therapy for Depression*:** Z. V. Segal, J. M. G. Williams, J. D. Teasdale, and J. Kabat-Zinn, *Mindfulness-Based Cognitive Therapy for Depression* (New York: Guilford Press, 2002).

classic examples of chronic "whole body" stressors: M. Prince, V. Patel, S. Saxena, et al., "No Health Without Mental Health," *Lancet* 370, no. 9590 (2007): 859–77.

we showed visual cues (pictures): C. Westbrook J. D. Creswell, G. Tabibnia, E.

Julson, H. Kober, and H. A. Tindle, "Mindful Attention Reduces Neural and Self-Reported Cue-Induced Craving in Smokers," *Social Cognitive and Affective Neuroscience* (November 22, 2011).

Intimacy with God: An Introduction to Centering Prayer: T. Keating, *Intimacy with God: An Introduction to Centering Prayer* (Danvers, MA: Crossroad Publishing Company, 2009).

to train health professionals in this practice: D. Bresler and M. Rossman, co-founders, *Academy for Guided Imagery,* March 13, 2006, www.academyforguided imagery.com; see also: D. Bresler and M. Rossman, *Guided Imagery Program: Breaking the Smoking Habit,* American Specialty Health, 2002.

psychologists Dr. William Miller and Dr. Stephen Rollnick: W. R. Miller and S. Rollnick, *Motivational Interviewing: Preparing People for Change,* 2nd ed. (New York: The Guildford Press, 2002).

start living that way *now*: J. T. Wilkins, H. Ning, L. Zhao, A. R. Dyer, D. M. Lloyd-Jones, "Lifetime Risk and Years Lived Free of Total Cardiovascular Disease." *JAMA: Journal of the American Medi-*

cal Association 308, no. 17 (2012): 1795–801.

Chapter 5: The Savvy Outlook Traveler 3

The Undefeated Mind: On the Science of Constructing an Indestructible Self: A. Lickerman, *The Undefeated Mind: On the Science of Constructing an Indestructible Self* (Deerfield Beach: Health Communications Inc., 2012).

psychology researcher and author of *Positivity*: B. Fredrickson, *Positivity: Groundbreaking Research Reveals How to Embrace the Hidden Strength of Positive Emotions, Overcome Negativity, and Thrive* (New York: MJF Books, 2012).

new neurons in the adult brain, termed *neurogenesis*: A. C. Pereira, D. E. Huddleston, A. M. Brickman, et al., "An In Vivo Correlate of Exercise-Induced Neurogenesis in the Adult Dentate Gyrus," *PNAS: Proceedings of the National Academy of Sciences of the United States of America* 104, no. 13 (2007): 5638–43.

benefits of exercise is the 2008 book *Spark*: J. J. Ratey, *Spark: The Revolutionary New Science of Exercise and the Brain*

(New York: Little, Brown and Company, 2008).

2011 study led by Dr. Kirk Erickson: K. I. Erickson, M. W. Voss, R. S. Prakash, et al., "Exercise Training Increases Size of Hippocampus and Improves Memory," *PNAS: Proceedings of the National Academy of Sciences* 108, no. 7 (2011): 3017–22.

your pancreas needs a good night's sleep, too: K. L. Knutson, K. Spiegel, P. Penev, and E. Van Cauter, "The Metabolic Consequences of Sleep Deprivation," *Sleep Med Reviews* 11, no 3. (2007): 163–78.

In one recent study of sleep restriction: J. L. Broussard, D. A. Ehrmann, E. Van Cauter, E. Tasali, and M. J. Brady, "Impaired Insulin Signaling in Human Adipocytes After Experimental Sleep Restriction: A Randomized, Crossover Study," *Annals of Internal Medicine* 157, no. 8 (2012): 549–57.

author Susan Cain is right: S. Cain and K. Mazur, *Quiet: The Power of Introverts in a World That Can't Stop Talking* (Thorndike, ME: Center Point Pub, 2012).

pass through social networks like propagating waves: J. H. Fowler and

N. A. Christakis, "Dynamic Spread of Happiness in a Large Social Network: Longitudinal Analysis over 20 Years in the Framingham Heart Study," *BMJ* 337 (2008): a2338; see also: N. A. Christakis and J. H. Fowler, "The Collective Dynamics of Smoking in a Large Social Network," *New England Journal of Medicine* 358, no. 21 (2008): 2249–58; and N. A. Christakis, "Social Networks and Collateral Health Effects," *BMJ* 329, no. 7459 (2004): 184–85.

"It's so peaceful": A. Fuller, "In the Shadow of Wounded Knee," *National Geographic,* August 2012.

***Urban Place: Reconnecting with the Natural World*:** P. F. Bartlett, *Urban Place: Reconnecting with the Natural World* (Cambridge, MA: MIT Press, 2005).

the gap between rich and poor in the risk of death was much greater: R. Mitchell and F. Popham, "Effect of Exposure to Natural Environment on Health Inequalities: An Observational Population Study," *Lancet* 372, no. 9650 (2008): 1655–60.

"I touch the soil and bad things go away": C. Newman, "Russian Summer," *National Geographic,* July 2012.

oxytocin is related to traits such as optimism: S. Saphire-Bernstein, B. M. Way, H. S. Kim, D. K. Sherman, and S. E. Taylor, "Oxytocin Receptor Gene (OXTR) Is Related to Psychological Resources," *Proceedings of the National Academy of Sciences of the United States of America* 108, no. 37 (2011): 15118–22.

known for its role in parent-child bonding: J. A. Bartz, J. Zaki, N. Bolger, et al., "Oxytocin Selectively Improves Empathic Accuracy," *Psychological Science* 21, no. 10 (2010): 1426–28.

have produced evidence to support this view: R. R. McCrae and P. T. Costa, "The Stability of Personality: Observations and Evaluations," *Current Directions in Psychological Science* 3, no. 6 (1994): 173–75; see also: P. T. Costa, J. H. Herbst, R. R. McCrae, and I. C. Siegler, "Personality at Midlife: Stability, Intrinsic Maturation, and Response to Life Events," *Assessment* 7, no. 4 (2000): 365–78.

our personalities continue to grow and change with us: B. W. Roberts, K. E. Walton, W. Viechtbauer, "Patterns of Mean-level Change in Personality Traits Across the Life Course: A Meta-analysis of Longitudinal Studies," *Psychological Bulletin* 132, no. 1 (2006): 1–25.

Mindset: The New Psychology of Success: C. S. Dweck, *Mindset: The New Psychology of Success* (New York: Random House, 2006).

personalities and their capacity for change: J. Aronson, C. Fried, and C. Good, "Reducing the Effects of Stereotype Threat on African American College Students by Shaping Theories of Intelligence," *Journal of Experimental Social Psychology* 38, no. 2 (2002): 113–25.

". . . and when they are, so too is personality": C. S. Dweck, "Can Personality Be Changed?: The Role of Beliefs in Personality and Change," *Current Directions in Psychological Science* 17, no. 6 (2008): 394.

"Broaden and Build": B. L. Fredrickson, "The Role of Positive Emotions in Positive Psychology. The Broaden-and-Build Theory of Positive Emotions," *American Psychologist* 56, no. 3 (2001): 218–26.

a clinical instructor at Harvard Medical School, and coeditor of *Wisdom and Compassion in Psychotherapy*: C. K. Germer and R. D. Siegel, *Wisdom and Compassion in Psychotherapy: Deepening*

Mindfulness in Clinical Practice (New York: Guilford Press, 2012), pp. xxiii, 407; see also: C. K. Germer, R. D. Siegel, and P. R. Fulton, *Mindfulness and Psychotherapy* (New York: Guilford Press, 2005); and C. K. Germer and S. Salzberg, *The Mindful Path to Self-Compassion: Freeing Yourself from Destructive Thoughts and Emotions* (New York: Guilford Press, 2009), pp. xiv, 306.

The Compassionate Mind: A New Approach to Life's Challenges: P. Gilbert, *The Compassionate Mind: A New Approach to Life's Challenges* (Oakland, CA: New Harbinger Publications, 2009).

Chapter 7: Looking Up Is Especially Important When You're Down

8 percent had three or more risk factors: Tindle, et al. "Psychological Attitudes and Risk of CHD."

women age 45 to 75 (and of different races): Berry, et al., "Lifetime Risks of Cardiovascular Disease."

pessimism was the better predictor of heart attack and death: H. A. Tindle, C. Y., K. A. Matthews, et al. "Is Trait Optimism or Pessimism More Important for Incident CHD and Mortality?" *Psy-*

chosomatic Medicine 73 (2010): A81–A82.

pessimism affected the postsurgical course of these patients: Tindle, et al., "Optimism, Response to Treatment of Depression."

prescriptions with the physician when appropriate: B. L. Rollman, B. H. Belnap, M. S. LeMenager, et al., "Telephone-Delivered Collaborative Care for Treating Post-CABG Depression: A Randomized Controlled Trial," *JAMA: Journal of the American Medical Association* 302, no. 19 (2009): 2095–103; see also: B. L. Rollman, B. H. Belnap, M. S. LeMenager, S. Mazumdar, H. C. Schulberg, and C. F. Reynolds 3rd, "The Bypassing the Blues Treatment Protocol: Stepped Collaborative Care for Treating Post-CABG Depression," *Psychosomatic Medicine* 71, no. 2 (2009): 217–30.

deadly combination of diabetes and obesity: F. Kaufman, *Diabesity: The Obesity-Diabetes Epidemic That Threatens America — And What We Must Do to Stop It* (New York: Random House, 2005).

for her discoveries that broken chromosomes were implicated in leukemias: J. D. Rowley, "Identification of a Translocation with Quinacrine Fluorescence in a Patient with Acute Leukemia," *Annales de Génétique* 16, no. 2 (1973): 109–12; see also: J. D. Rowley, "Letter: A New Consistent Chromosomal Abnormality in Chronic Myelogenous Leukaemia Identified by Quinacrine Fluorescence and Giemsa Staining," *Nature* 243, no. 5405 (1973): 290–93; J. D. Rowley, "Chromosomal Patterns in Myelocytic Leukemia," *New England Journal of Medicine* 289, no. 4 (1973): 220–21; J. D. Rowley, "Acquired Trisomy 9," *Lancet* 2, no. 7825 (1973): 390; and J. D. Rowley, "Letter: Deletions of Chromosome 7 in Haematological Disorders," *Lancet* 2, no. 7842 (1973): 1385–86.

confirming the existence of a third translocation: J. D. Rowley, H. M. Golomb, and C. Dougherty, "15/17 Translocation, a Consistent Chromosomal Change in Acute Promyelocytic Leukaemia," *Lancet* 1, no. 8010 (1977): 549–50; see also: H. M. Golomb, J. D. Rowley, J. W. Vardiman, J. R. Testa, and A. Butler,

" 'Microgranular' Acute Promyelocytic Leukemia: A Distinct Clinical, Ultrastructural, and Cytogenetic Entity," *Blood* 55, no. 2 (1980): 253–59.

Judith Anne Rice (and described in her book of the same name): J. A. Rice, *The Kindness Curriculum: Introducing Young Children to Loving Values* (St. Paul, MN: Redleaf Press, 1995).

results of this project are expected in the near future: D. Erickson, "Investigating Healthy Minds: Preschool Study Seeks to Teach Kindness," *Wisconsin State Journal* May 18, 2011: http://host.madison .com/news/local/health_med_fit/investigat ing-healthy-minds-preschool-study-seeks-to-teach-kindness/article_f7861ede-8194-11e0-903d-001cc4c002e0.html (accessed 11/15/12).

compared with people who received standard cardiac advice: M. Friedman, C. E. Thoresen, J. J. Gill, et al., "Feasibility of Altering Type A Behavior Pattern After Myocardial Infarction. Recurrent Coronary Prevention Project Study: Methods, Baseline Results and Preliminary Findings" *Circulation* 66, no. 1 (1982): 83–92.

"and tries to reduce obesity in the

population": T. A. Farley, "The Role of Government in Preventing Excess Calorie Consumption: The Example of New York City," *JAMA: Journal of the American Medical Association* 308, no. 11 (2012): 1093–94; see also: G. P. Rodgers and F. S. Collins, "The Next Generation of Obesity Research: No Time to Waste," *JAMA: Journal of the American Medical Association* 308, no. 11 (2012): 1095–96.

his book *The Optimistic Child*: Seligman, et al., *The Optimistic Child*.

and found some surprising results: K. A. Robb, A. E. Simon, and J. Wardle, "Socioeconomic Disparities in Optimism and Pessimism," *International Journal of Behavioral Medicine* 16, no. 4 (2009): 331–38.

a greater sense of well-being: J. Ludwig, G. J. Duncan, L. A. Gennetian, et al., "Neighborhood Effects on the Long-Term Well-Being of Low-Income Adults," *Science* 337, no. 6101 (2012): 1505–10.

trappings of low SES may do us biological harm: K. A. Matthews, L. C. Gallo, and S. E. Taylor, "Are Psychosocial Factors Mediators of Socioeconomic Status and Health Connections? A Progress Report and Blueprint for the Future," *An-*

nals of the New York Academy of Sciences 1186 (2010): 146–73.

overactive stress biology as "weathering": "Weathering the Storm," *Miller-McCune,* June 15, 2009; see also: A. T. Geronimus, M. Hicken, D. Keene, and J. Bound, " 'Weathering' and Age Patterns of Allostatic Load Scores Among Blacks and Whites in the United States," *American Journal of Public Health* 96, no. 5 (2006): 826–33.

***The Status Syndrome: How Social Standing Affects our Health and Longevity*:** M. G. Marmot, "Status Syndrome: A Challenge to Medicine," *JAMA: Journal of the American Medical Association* 295, no. 11 (2006): 1304–7; see also: M. G. Marmot, *The Status Syndrome: How Social Standing Affects Our Health and Longevity* (New York: Times Books, 2004); and M. G. Marmot, "Understanding Social Inequalities in Health," *Perspectives in Biology and Medicine* 46, no. 3 (Suppl.) (2003): S9–S23.

articulated in 2008: M. Marmot, S. Friel, R. Bell, et al., "Closing the Gap in a Generation: Health Equity Through Action on the Social Determinants of Health" *Lancet* 372 (2008): 1661–69.

more recently in the 2012 summary: M. Marmot, J. Allen, R. Bell, et al., "WHO European Review of Social Determinants of Health and the Health Divide," *Lancet* 380, no. 9846 (2012): 1011–29.

SES, influences our risk of cardiovascular disease and death: A. V. Diez Roux and C. Mair, "Neighborhoods and Health," *Annals of the New York Academy of Sciences* 1186, no. 1 (2010): 125–45; see also: C. Mair, A. V. Diez Roux, M. Shen, et al., "Cross-Sectional and Longitudinal Associations of Neighborhood Cohesion and Stressors with Depressive Symptoms in the Multiethnic Study of Atherosclerosis," *Annals of Epidemiology* 19, no. 1 (2009): 49–57; and A. V. Diez Roux, S. S. Merkin, D. Arnett, et al., "Neighborhood of Residence and Incidence of Coronary Heart Disease," *New England Journal of Medicine* 345, no. 2 (2001): 99–106.

"quality of neighborhoods and communal life": M. Marmot, "Inequalities in Health," NEJM: *New England Journal of Medicine* 345, no. 99 (2001): 106–7.

***I Beat the Odds: From Homelessness to* The Blind Side *and Beyond*:** M. Oher and D. Yaeger, *I Beat the Odds: From*

Homelessness to The Blind Side *and Beyond* (New York: Gotham Books, 2011).

"the mind-set I had to succeed, with or without anyone's help": Ibid, p. 9.

what Michael endured barrage the body and mind: J. P. Shonkoff and A. S. Garner, "The Lifelong Effects of Early Childhood Adversity and Toxic Stress," *Pediatrics* 129, no. 1 (2012): e232–e46; see also: A. S. Garner and J. P. Shonkoff, "Early Childhood Adversity, Toxic Stress, and the Role of the Pediatrician: Translating Developmental Science into Lifelong Health," *Pediatrics* 129, no. 1 (2012): e224–e31.

"then we basically lose a reason to live": Oher, *I Beat the Odds,* p. 68.

INDEX